Where To From Here? Examining Conflict-Related and Relational Interaction Trauma

At the Interface/Probing the Boundaries

VOLUME 98

The titles published in this series are listed at *brill.com/aipb*

Where To From Here? Examining Conflict-Related and Relational Interaction Trauma

Edited by

Elspeth McInnes and Anka D. Mason

TUTA SUB AEGIDE PALLAS · 1683 ·

BRILL
RODOPI

LEIDEN | BOSTON

Cover illustration: “Sunrise seagull silhouette”. Photographer: Alex Wigan (@alwig64). Retrieved via Unsplash.

The Library of Congress Cataloging-in-Publication Data is available online at http://catalog.loc.gov
LC record available at http://lccn.loc.gov/2019902218

Typeface for the Latin, Greek, and Cyrillic scripts: “Brill”. See and download: brill.com/brill-typeface.

ISSN 1570-7113
ISBN 978-90-04-35080-9 (paperback)
ISBN 978-90-04-39757-6 (e-book)

This book is printed on acid-free paper and produced in a sustainable manner.

Contents

Notes on Contributors

Kim M. Anderson

PhD LCSW is a Professor of Social Work and Public Affairs at the University of Central Florida, USA. As highlighted in her book, *Enhancing Resilience in Survivors Family Violence* (Anderson, 2010), her scholarship bridges gaps between theory and practice by offering conceptual frameworks that captures the interplay of trauma and resilience for survivors of family violence and mental health practitioners.

Lyn Barnes

is a senior lecturer in journalism at Auckland University of Technology, New Zealand. Her PhD thesis focused on trauma journalism and journalists who deal with trauma day-to-day.

Catherine Ann Collins

is a Professor of Rhetoric at Willamette University in Salem, Oregon USA. She teaches and does research in trauma and narrative theory, visual and commemorative rhetoric, and the rhetoric of war.

Fran S. Danis

PhD is Associate Professor Emeritus of Social Work at the University of Texas – Arlington, USA. Her research includes self-efficacy of practitioners, resiliency of abuse survivors and their adult daughters, and developing coordinated community responses to crime victims. Currently, she is a researcher and evaluator for gender justice.

Stefanie Marie Margarete Dinkelbach

PhD is an independent artist, film-maker and scholar based in Cork, Ireland. She recently completed a practice-based doctorate in film which involved producing *Das Vermächtnis* (*The Legacy*), an audio-visual reflection on collective memory that pays tribute to the victims of the Holocaust.

Lyda Eleftheriou

is a Lecturer in English and the Induction Programme Leader at UNICAF University. Her research interests lie in the realms of postcolonial literature, psychoanalytic theory and memory studies. She is currently pursuing her PhD at University of Cyprus, focusing on South Asian Partition Fiction in English.

Kirsten Havig

PhD, MSW is an Assistant Professor of Social Work at The University of Wyoming, USA. Her research focuses on violence against women; the commercial sexual exploitation of children; trauma, resilience, and posttraumatic growth; and social justice pedagogy in social work education. Prior to working in higher education she was a Licensed Clinical Social Worker who practiced with child welfare- and justice-involved youth, and survivors of sexual trauma.

Anka D. Mason

is an independent human rights legal scholar and activist. Her work focuses on issues of body, gender, violence, and rights advocacy within conflict and post-conflict communities.

Elspeth McInnes

BA Hons 1 PhD is a sociologist and Associate Professor in the School of Education at the University of South Australia. Her teaching and research is focused on educator knowledge of family violence and abuse, parental separation and divorce and the social policies addressing these issues.

Joan Simalchik

teaches in the Historical Studies Department, University of Toronto Mississauga, where she is the Program Coordinator for Women and Gender Studies. Joan served as the founding executive director of the Canadian Centre for Victims of Torture.

Stephanie Y. Tam

is an independent writer, researcher and producer. She completed an MSc in Evidence-Based Social Intervention and an MSt in World Literatures in the Department of English Language and Literature at the University of Oxford as a Daniel M. Sachs Scholar. Her research interests include trauma theory, narrative therapy, postcolonial and migration studies and, the role of fantasy in memory reconstruction, which she also explores in her own creative work.

Rana Tayara

a native of Lebanon, has witnessed the effects of war on the Lebanese children and adolescents. After graduating with a Ph.D. in Psychology from the University of York UK, she has published several articles on the well-being of adults and adolescents in post conflict environments.

Introduction: Rupture, Recovery and Spaces Between

Anka D. Mason

> Speaking of Trauma
> Words were invented to speak of the visible, not to speak of the invisible. Thus, all expressions of an experience are going to be metaphoric [and, therefore,] we are confined to poetry.[1]
>
> Author's Translation

∵

With no agreed upon definition concerning the word *trauma* as applied to mentally debilitating ruptures that create intense fear, anxiety and suffering, we are left with the standard definition from the Greek for *wound*. It is often the case in collective, interdisciplinary writings such as these, therefore, that writers attempt, though the sharing of the empirical observations in the psychosocial realm, explorations of literary works and other genres of expression, to capture meaning and make sense of this term *trauma*. Perhaps by borrowing again from vocabulary coined originally for medical interventions, a summary of what is contained herein may be achieved. And in connection to wounding (*trauma*) the borrowed term is *intention*. The adaptation of this term with the medical connotation in relation to this collection of writings allows multiple meanings and analogies to emerge for the reader. Here the word *intention* connotes the plan for healing.[2] With this meaning, we may consider the ways that a 'clear vision of a desired outcome,'[3] Chopra's definition for intention in

1 Leili Anvar, '*La révélation au desert*: An interview with Éric-Emmanuel Schmitt (*La nuit de feu*),' *Les raciness du ciel*, podcast audio, 6 September 2015, http://www.franceculture.fr/emissions/les-racines-du-ciel/la-revelation-au-desert.

2 Marianne Saunorus Baird, *Manual of Critical Care Nursing: Nursing Interventions and Collaborative Management*, 7th ed., (St. Louis: Elsevier Health Sciences, 2015), 183, viewed 13 November 2015, http://ccn.aacnjournals.org/content/37/1/81.full.

3 Deepak Chopra, *Meditation Experience*, podcast audio, 22 November 2015, https://chopracentermeditation.com/experience.

 | DOI:10.1163/9789004397576_002

relation to personal power of the self as consciously expressed, implies decision making processes, judgment, awareness toward healing.

Primary Intention-the Healing of an Incised Wound by Direct Union of Skin Edges without Granulations[4]

Where does one find 'edges' of psychological wounds? Perhaps the edges are located in with generations that succeed those that lived the original trauma or traumatic event or the survivors who bore witness to the original trauma. It may be that the contours of the wound(s) are in the memories of the time before the wound(ing) and the anticipation of safer, better future. This could be what we discover through literary works that attempt to mediate a particular traumatic event or events. This is the medium of inquiry into trauma found in *Lyda Eleftheriou*'s chapter (The Present and the Future of the Past: The Lasting Gift of the Indian Partition to its Descendants) and *Stephanie Y. Tam*'s chapter (Worlds after War: Negotiating the Art of Losing in J.R.R. Tolkien's *Lord of the Rings*).

Granulations are defined as the production of new connective tissue at the edges of the wound.[5] With a primary intervention, to close the wound without the granulations is to purposefully bypass this auto-healing process. In consideration of trauma in theory and practice, this brings to mind the question of whether this is sometimes the more preferable route. This brings to mind as well, in the case of the flesh, the body's natural inclination toward healing, toward wound closure. Is this necessarily the case with psychological wounds? Or, is it the case that one must purposefully intend (in the non-medical sense of the word) toward healing—that one must *want* to heal? The Purposeful, conscious intervention is what we see in the writings of *Kim M. Anderson, Kristen Havig and Fran S. Danis* (Adult Daughters of Intimate Partner Violence Survivors: From Childhood Powerlessness to Adult Empowerment) and *Catherine Ann Collins* (Living with Someone Both Here and Gone: Trauma and Dementia).

Language as the Granulation of Healing in Trauma

The role of language and perception in relation to intention as applied here (a plan for healing) emerges as somewhat of a challenge when we consider

4 Baird, *Manual of Critical Care Nursing*, 183–184.

5 Ibid., 185.

questions of what to do when language for traumatic events shifts in form and shows up as art as in *Elspeth McInnes'* chapter (Young Children's Drawings After Sexual Abuse: Disclosure and Recovery). Equally important for consideration is the way that public perception of traumas and traumatic events are shaped by those reporting on these events and how these reporters of trauma are affected or wounded, a topic explored by *Lyn Barnes* (The Resilient Journalist: Making Dollars and Sense).

Secondary Intention—the Wound Is Left Open and Heals on Its Own through the Formation of Granulations[6]

Are public, social rituals, disclosures, and acts of justice seeking different types of granulations in the instance and aftermath of trauma? Are these the acts that become the new blood vessels and flesh that join the past and present toward future that is existence within a healed state? This may be just the lens necessary to consider the collective trauma and aftermath of oppression, torture, and rape of mass conflict settings as explored by *Joan Simalchik* (The Public Dimension of Privatized Trauma: Impact and Response) and *Anka D. Mason* (Unpacking Male Sexualized Trauma: Rights and Resistance from a Feminist Perspective).

Third Intention—the Wound Is Left Open for a Number of Days and Then Closed If Found to Be Clean[7]

Perhaps the most difficult aspect in speaking of trauma as wound is in considering how the healing process may be elusive for many where the harm and its effects generally remain invisible and therefore difficult measure or to put into words. The particular challenges of locating and measuring the harmful and in many cases long-lasting effects of trauma are the subject of investigations found in *Rana Tayara's* piece (Resiliency, a Mediator Between War Experience and Aggressive Behaviour) and *Stefanie Marie Margarete Dinklebach*'s piece (Finding the Way Home: An Interdisciplinary Perspective on Trauma and Trauma Resolution Practices).

---

6 Ibid., 185.

7 Encyclopaedia Britannica Online, *Third Intention*, viewed 13 November 2016, http://global.britannica.com/science/third-intention.

Wounds, Healing, Resilience as Sites of Contestation

Examining the traumatic with a sense of the constraints of language allows us to then begin to define and even redefine with a sense of liberty though the use of metaphor and poetry. This freedom, however, exposes one of the greater challenges to understanding trauma and the traumatic: the fact that one cannot be brought fully into the subjective, sensorial experience of another. Moreover, and as discussed throughout the volume, we are left to what can be observed in the realm of the physical and our perceptions and cognitions of the same in order to render our meaning(s). We are left with trying to make *sense* through *resonance* as used to indicate *echo* and *sympathy*. Resonance will be elaborated further through subjective and intersubjective filters of self, identity, and narrative. With this in mind, how then does one imagine the concept of resilience as applied to the varied and multifaceted subjects and approaches found within this volume? Is *resilience* to be understood as the "capacity to withstand repeated shocks," as understood and connoted from the perspective of physics? Or, as the more nuanced definitions applied to the psychosocial fields of study allow, are we to understand resilience as a person's capacity or cope, to live (deal) with, to survive? Is it proper to apply this particular term in speaking of the traumatic and the processes of healing? Perhaps the answers to these questions lie in what we, as survivors, practitioners, support networks, and the generally concern intend with our thoughts, words, and actions when aiding or being of service to those dealing with unspeakable anguish of experiences without words, meaning, or sense.

Speaking to and for the Silent Wounded and the Permanently Silenced

One of the many aims of this volume and of its contributors is to give voice to issues around trauma that are often left on the margins of discourses that may be too technical in nature or too narrow in scope to allow for discussions of themes addressed herein. It is hoped, however, that readers of this volume will consider as well those whose voices are not present: the wilfully and the unwillingly silent, the disappeared, and the *non-survivors* of trauma. This last group includes both those that have lost their lives and those that have taken their own lives. As one of the authors of this volume insisted during the conference that was the impetus for this volume, when speaking of resilience, we must also consider its opposite when applying it to trauma and the traumatic.

We must remember, she insisted, that there are many for whom the capacity to be resilient, to cope, to manage, to survive in the aftermath of trauma is simply too overwhelming.[8] Indeed, those lost to trauma and traumatic events should be considered in our reading and contemplation of this volume and in the discussions that follow. Resilience as a term is perhaps then best applied to the survivors of this loss; resonance, as discussed above, to the impressions that emerge for those left behind; and the consideration of worthiness of metaphor and poetry, in this instance, enlarged. Perhaps, then, in the readings that follow one should hold in mind a conceptualisation of wounds as processes of opening, re-layering (with or without intentions and interventions), and healing as an intention that unfolds without contours, but within the confines of metaphor and poetry.

Bibliography

Anvar, Leili. '*La révélation au desert*: An interview with Éric-Emmanuel Schmitt (*La nuit de feu*).' *Les raciness du ciel*. Podcast audio. 6 September 2015. http://www.franceculture.fr/emissions/les-racines-du-ciel/la-revelation-au-desert.

Baird, Marianne Saunorus. *Manual of Critical Care Nursing: Nursing Interventions and Collaborative Management*, 7th edition. St. Louis: Elsevier Health Sciences, 2015. Viewed online 13 November 2015. http://ccn.aacnjournals.org/content/37/1/81.full

Chopra, Deepak. *Meditation Experience*. Podcast Audio. 22 November 2015. https://chopracentermeditation.com/experience.

Encyclopaedia Britannica Online. *Third Intention*. Viewed 13 November 2016. http://global.britannica.com/science/third-intention.

8 Author Stefanie Marie Margarete Dinklebach's commentary on the use of the word *resilience* in connection with emotion and mental trauma. (paper presented at the Inter-Disciplinary. Net, 4th Global Conference, Trauma: Practice and Theory, Prague, Czech Republic, 22 March–25 March 2014), notes on file with author.

CHAPTER 1

Adult Daughters of Intimate Partner Violence Survivors: from Childhood Powerlessness to Adult Empowerment

Kim M. Anderson, Kirsten Havig and Fran S. Danis

Abstract

This chapter reports on a qualitative study that addresses the recovery process for adult daughters (N = 15) of intimate partner violence (IPV) survivors. Through the use of the grounded theory method, participants' recovery was found to include a journey of self-discovery (starting with childhood in a violent home) often characterized by confusion and undeserved guilt, always distinguished by powerlessness, to a state of personal power and the possibility of choice (in adulthood). Three progressive, yet not mutually exclusive, stages were germane to transforming childhood powerlessness into adult empowerment: deconstruction of childhood beliefs, reformation of childhood misperceptions, and transcendence of childhood experiences. Implications for helping professionals and adult daughters of abuse survivors include providing a conceptual framework to better understand the positive changes individuals make to recover from childhood exposure to domestic violence.

Keywords

children exposed to domestic violence – child witnesses – intimate partner violence – recovery

Children do not have to experience violence directly to suffer from it. Because of its abusive and often prolonged nature, children exposed to their mothers' Intimate Partner Violence (IPV) present with stressors that often go beyond the adaptive capacities of most children and may produce long-lasting effects. Witnessing violent acts and enduring a family environment characterized by control, fear, and powerlessness often negatively impacts

 | DOI:10.1163/9789004397576_003

children's adaptive abilities, social functioning, emotional well-being, and physical health.[1] Children are highly affected by exposure to violence involving people close to them; consequently, many may carry a psychological price that continues to be paid into adulthood.[2]

Although research indicates that witnessing inter-parental violence as a child is related to long-term consequences, there remains a dearth of knowledge in regard to the recovery process for this population. Studies, such as the Adverse Childhood Experiences (ACES),[3] confirm the negative impact on adults who as children were exposed to violence and other traumatic experiences. Although we are becoming more knowledgeable in all areas of childhood trauma, minimal research has been undertaken in regard to adult recovery for child witnesses. 'Most research on the adult effects of abuse have focused on sexual and physical abuse, and far less is known about how witnessing domestic violence as a child affects adult women in particular.'[4] This chapter reports on a qualitative study that addresses this gap to better understand and detail the recovery process for adult daughters of IPV survivors.

1 Sibylle Artz, Margaret A. Jackson, Katherine R. Rossiter, Alicia Nijdam-Jones, István Géczy and Sheila Porteous, 'A Comprehensive Review of the Literature on the Impact of Exposure to Intimate Partner Violence on Children and Youth,' *Journal of Child, Youth and Family Studies* 5.4 (2014): 493–587; Stephanie Holt, Helen Buckley and Sadhbh Whelan, 'The Impact of Exposure to Domestic Violence on Children and Young People: A Review of the Literature,' *Child Abuse and Neglect* 32 (2008): 797–810; Katie A. McLaughlin et al., 'Childhood Social Environment, Emotional Reactivity to Stress, and Mood and Anxiety Disorders across the Life Course,' *Depression and Anxiety* 27 (2010): 1087–1094.

2 Allison N. Ponce, Michelle K. Williams and George J. Allen, 'Experience of Maltreatment as a Child and Acceptance of Violence in Adult Intimate Relationships: Mediating Effects of Distortions in Cognitive Schemas,' *Violence and Victims* 19.1 (2004): 97–108; Asa K. Cater, Laura E. Miller, Kathryn H. Howell, and Sandra A. Graham-Bermann, 'Childhood Exposure to Intimate Partner Violence and Adult Mental Health Problems: Relationships with Gender and Age of Exposure,' *Journal of Family Violence* 30 (2015): 875–886.

3 Valerie J. Edwards, Robert F. Anda, Vincent J. Felitti and Shanta R. Dube, 'Adverse Childhood Experiences and Health-Related Quality of Life as an Adult,' *Health Consequences of Abuse in the Family: A Clinical Guide for Evidence-Based Practice*, ed. K. A. Kendall-Tackett (Washington, DC: American Psychological Association, 2004), 81–94; Vincent J. Felitti et al., 'Relationship of Childhood Abuse and Household Dysfunction to Many of the Leading Causes of Death in Adults: The Adverse Childhood Experiences (ACE) Study,' *American Journal of Preventive Medicine* 14.4 (1998): 245–258.

4 Kimberly D. Becker, Jeffrey Stuewig and Laura A. McClosky, 'Traumatic Stress Symptoms of Women Exposed to Different Forms of Childhood Victimization and Intimate Partner Violence,' *Journal of Interpersonal Violence* 25.9 (2010): 1701.

1 Childhood Exposure to IPV: Challenges to the Recovery Process

Approximately fifteen million children are exposed to domestic violence each year with seven million living in families with severe partner violence.[5] Research findings indicate a link between IPV exposure and the development of symptomatology for children including behavioural problems such as conduct disorder,[6] physical aggression, hyperactivity, inattentiveness, impulsivity, destructiveness, and noncompliance.[7] Additionally, child victims may blame themselves for the violence and feel helpless to change their family situation thereby creating internalizing problems such as depression, anxiety, low self-esteem, and somatic complaints.[8] Children exposed to IPV have also been found to be at greater risk for co-occurring physical and sexual abuse.[9]

Social adjustment difficulties include poor peer relationships, academic problems, a lack of adaptive interpersonal attachments, and an increased likelihood that a child will become either a victim (often females) or perpetrator

5 Megan Bair-Merritt, Barry Zuckerman, Marilyn Augustyn, and Peter F. Cronholm, 'Silent victims – An Epidemic of Childhood Exposure to Domestic Violence,' The *New England Journal of Medicine* 369.18 (2013): 1673–1675; Renee McDonald, et al., 'Estimating the Number of American Children Living in Partner-Violent Families,' *Journal of Family Psychology*, 20.1 (2006): 137–142.

6 Kim M. Anderson and Eun-Jun Bang, 'Assessing PTSD and Resilience for Females who during Childhood were Exposed to Domestic Violence,' *Child and Family Social Work* 17.1 (2012): 55–65; Howard Meltzer et al., 'The Mental Health of Children who Witness Domestic Violence,' *Child and Family Social Work* 14 (2009): 491–501.

7 Gayla Margolin and Katrina A. Vickerman, 'Post-Traumatic Stress in Children and Adolescents Exposed to Family Violence: Overview and Issues,' *Couple and Family Psychology: Research and Practice* 1 (2011): 63–73; Judith M. McFarlane, Janet Y. Groff, Jennifer A. O'Brien and Kathy Watson, 'Behaviors of Children who are Exposed and Not Exposed to Intimate Partner Violence: An Analysis of 330 Black, White, and Hispanic Children,' *Pediatrics* 112 (2003): e202–e207; Judee E. Onyskiw, 'Domestic Violence and Children's Adjustment: A Review of Research,' *Journal of Emotional Abuse* 3 (2003): 11–45.

8 Katherine M. Kitzmann, Noni K. Gaylord, Aimee R. Holt and Erin D. Kenny, 'Child Witnesses to Domestic Violence: A Meta-Analytic Review,' *Journal of Consulting and Clinical Psychology* 71 (2003): 339–352; Matthew W. Reynolds et al., 'The Relationship between Gender, Depression, and Self-Esteem in Children who have Witnessed Domestic Violence,' *Child Abuse and Neglect* 25 (2001): 1201–1206.

9 Mariette Chartier, John R. Walker and Barbara Naimark, 'Seperate and Cumulative Effects of Adverse Childhood Experiences in Predicting Adult Health and Health Care Utilization,' *Child Abuse and Neglect* 34 (2010): 454–464; Francien Lamers-Winkelman, Agnes M. Willeman, and Margreet Visser, 'Adverse Childhood Experiences of Referred Children Exposed to Intimate Partner Violence: Consequences for Their Wellbeing,' *Child Abuse and Neglect* 36 (2012): 166–179.

(often males) of violence later in life.[10] Consequently, the intergenerational legacy of IPV is also evident.[11] While child witnesses include boys and girls, a few studies report gender differences regarding the impact of witnessing IPV.[12] Thus, exploring separately each gender's developmental trajectory allows for gender-based relevant discovery and explication of short- and long-term impacts.

The life trajectories of adults exposed to abuse of their mothers by male partners are receiving more attention. Research studies demonstrate the obstacles for adult daughters of abuse survivors to achieving successful psychosocial outcomes.[13] In comparison to non-exposed individuals, adult daughters experience greater depression,[14] anxiety,[15] drug abuse,[16] self-doubt,[17] distorted cognitive schemas, behaviour and learning problems,[18] obesity and other

10 Caroline M. Clements, Claire Oxtoby and Richard L. Ogle, 'Methodological Issues in Assessing Psychological Adjustment in Child Witnesses of Intimate Partner Violence,' *Trauma, Violence, and Abuse* 9.2 (2008): 114–127.

11 Jessica Holt and Wayne Gillespie, 'Intergenerational Transmission of Violence, Threatened Egoism, and Reciprocity: A Test of Multiple Psychosocial Factors Affecting Intimate Partner Violence,' *American Journal of Criminal Justice* 33.2 (2008): 252–266; Timothy O. Ireland and Caroline Smith, 'Living in Partner-Violent Families: Developmental Links to Antisocial Behaviour and Relationship Violence,' *Journal of Youth and Adolescence* 38 (2009): 323–339.

12 Sarah Evans, Corrie Davies and David DiLillo, 'Exposure to Domestic Violence: A Meta-Analysis of Child and Adolescent Outcomes,' *Aggression and Violent Behaviour* 13.2 (2008): 131–140; Abigail A. Fagan and Emily M. Wright, 'Gender Differences in the Effects of Exposure to Intimate Partner Violence on Adolescent Violence and Drug Use,' *Child Abuse and Neglect* 35.7 (2011): 543–550; Veronica M. Herrera and Laura A. McCloskey, 'Gender Differences in the Risk for Delinquency among Youth Exposed to Family Violence,' *Child Abuse and Neglect* 25 (2001): 1037–1051.

13 Staci L. Suzuki, Robert Geffner and Steven F. Bucky, 'The Experiences of Adults Exposed to Intimate Partner Violence as Children: An Exploratory Qualitative Study of Resilience and Protective Factors,' *Journal of Emotional Abuse* 8.1/2 (2008): 103–121.

14 David Russell, Kristen W. Springer and Emily A. Greenfield, 'Witnessing Domestic Abuse in Childhood as an Independent Risk Factor for Depressive Symptoms in Adulthood,' *Child Abuse and Neglect* 34 (2010): 448–453.

15 Katie A. McLaughlin et al., 'Childhood Social Environment, Emotional Reactivity to Stress, and Mood and Anxiety Disorders across the Life Course,' *Depression and Anxiety* 27 (2010): 1087–1094.

16 Fagan and Wright, 'Gender Differences in the Effects of Exposure to Intimate Partner Violence on Adolescent Violence and Drug Use,' 543–550.

17 Michelle Moon, 'Retrospective Reports of Interparental Abuse by Adult Children from Intact Families,' *Journal of Interpersonal Violence* 15.12 (2000): 1323–1331.

18 Nadine J. Burke, Julia L. Hellman, Brandon G. Scott, Carl F. Weems and Victor G. Carrion, 'The Impact of Adverse Childhood Experiences on an Urban Pediatric Population,' *Child Abuse and Neglect* 35 (2011): 408–413.

major health problems,[19] and intimate partner violence.[20] Furthermore, childhood exposure to IPV has been found to create as much or more chronic psychological stress (i.e., PTSD, social avoidance, traumatic distress) than either childhood sexual or physical abuse for adult daughters.[21] These studies underscore the challenges to recovery for adult daughters. In addition to inquiry of negative impacts, more study is necessary that examines individuals' abilities to adapt, reorganize, and regenerate in the midst of recovery. Exploring how individuals prevail in the aftermath of violence and traumatic events remains a relatively new area of inquiry.[22]

2 Theoretical Framework: Constructivist Self-Development Theory

Constructivist Self-Development Theory (CSDT) provides the conceptual backdrop for this study. It offers a useful theoretical lens for recognizing and explaining that traumatic events like exposure to IPV during childhood can produce both negative and positive consequences for the affected individual.[23] Throughout one's life trajectory, newly developed competencies as well as problems may emerge. In trauma recovery, growth and pain are not necessarily opposites, but instead are different aspects of the overall experience of coping

19 Shanta R. Dube et al., 'Exposure to Abuse, Neglect, and Household Dysfunction among Adults who Witnessed Intimate Partner Violence as Children: Implications for Health and Social Services,' *Violence and Victims* 17.1 (2002): 3–17.

20 Azmaira H. Maker, Markus Kemmelmeier and Christopher Peterson, 'Long-Term Psychological Consequences in Women of Witnessing Parental Physical Conflict and Experiencing Abuse in Childhood,' *Journal of Interpersonal Violence* 13.5 (1998): 574–589.

21 Kimberly D. Becker, Jeffrey Stuewig and Laura A. McClosky, 'Traumatic Stress Symptoms of Women Exposed to Different Forms of Childhood Victimization and Intimate Partner Violence,' *Journal of Interpersonal Violence* 25.9 (2010): 1699–1715; Corrie A. Davies, David DiLillo and Isaac G. Martinez, 'Isolating Adult Psychological Correlates of Witnessing Parental Violence: Findings from a Predominantly Latina Sample,' *Journal of Family Violence* 19.6 (2004): 377–385.

22 Carolyn M. Aldwin and Michael R. Levenson, 'Posttraumatic Growth: Developmental Perspective,' *Psychological Inquiry* 15.1 (2004): 19–22; Becker, Stuewig, McClosky, 'Traumatic Stress Symptoms of Women Exposed to Different Forms of Childhood Victimization and Intimate Partner Violence,' *Journal of Interpersonal Violence* 25.9 (2010): 1699–1715; Kathryn H. Howell and Laura E. Miller-Graff, 'Protective Factors Associated with Resilient Functioning in Young Adulthood after Childhood Exposure to Violence,' *Child Abuse and Neglect* 38.12 (2014): 1985–1994.

23 Karen W. Saakvitne, Howard Tennen and Glen Affleck, 'Exploring Thriving in the Context of Clinical Trauma Theory: Constructivist Self Development Theory,' *Journal of Social Issues* 54.2 (1998): 279–299.

and adjustment. Trauma can disrupt individuals' views of themselves, relationships with others, as well as their core assumptions. Yet according to CSDT, confronting these disruptions may also promote expanded perspectives, new ways of coping, and the development of additional personal and social resources.[24]

More information is needed regarding the trauma experience as a vehicle for understanding how daughters of abused mothers alter childhood beliefs influenced by IPV and shape their adult identities. CSDT provides a context to better understand the impact of cognitive schemas that shape perceptions of the self, others, and the future. Calhoun and Tedeschi underscore how the reconstruction of meaning is necessary because trauma works by threatening or dismantling the individual's views of the self and the world; this process is anchored in the meaning that one attributes to the traumatic incident as well as in how one views oneself and the world.[25] It is constructivist in that individuals build and shape their own realities rooted in cognitive processes and contextualized by the environment; it is also a continual process as individuals develop.

The current study examined in more detail how in adulthood daughters transform childhood perceptions of powerlessness, through a deeper understanding of the political nature of abuse, to adult schemas of empowerment. CSDT provided a theoretical lens that illuminated this process. The findings, consistent with a feminist approach to working with IPV survivors, provide helping professionals and daughters with conceptual insights to better understand how in adulthood individuals reconfigure childhood assumptions and reconstruct identities of choice, pride, and potential.[26]

3 Method

The research aim was to qualitatively investigate adult daughters' recovery process in the aftermath of childhood exposure to IPV. For this study, recovery referred to ' a journey of self-discovery, a unique personal process of changing

24 Lawrence G. Calhoun and Richard G. Tedeschi, 'Beyond Recovery from Trauma: Implications for Clinical Practice and Research,' *Journal of Social Issues* 54.2 (1998): 357–371.

25 Ibid.

26 Angelique Jenney, Ramona Allagia, and Mark Niepage, 'The lie is that it's not going to get better: Narratives of resilience from childhood exposure to Intimate Partner Violence,' *International Journal of Child and Adolescent Resilience* 4.1 (2016): 64–76; Susan E. Roche and Gayle G. Wood, 'A Narrative Principle for Feminist Social Work with Survivors of Male Violence,' *Affilia* 20.4 (2005): 465–475.

one's attitudes, values, feelings and goals, and involves finding new meaning in life with or without the limitation caused by'[27] childhood exposure to IPV. Because the intent of this study was to illuminate the recovery process (i.e., conceptual dimensions and components) rather than outcomes, grounded theory was particularly suited as its purpose is to identify complex and hidden psychosocial processes.[28] This approach involved being 'immersed' in the world viewpoints of the participants and allowed for the influences of context on experience and meaning to be illuminated.

The study's two research questions were: 1) What is the process of recovery from childhood exposure to IPV among adult daughters? And, 2) What childhood beliefs and cognitive schemas about violence are altered in the recovery process and how does it impact the construction of identity in their own adult lives?

3.1 *Inclusion/Exclusion Criteria*

After approval by a university internal review board, participants were recruited through local newspaper advertisements in a small Midwestern city in the United States. Potential participants were screened over the telephone to explain the interview process and to determine whether they met sampling criteria. Although domestic violence also includes abuse by women against men and same-sex partners, the focus of this study was on the experience 'in which most children exposed to domestic violence find themselves, in a home where a man is committing a pattern of violence against an adult woman, who is most often the child's mother.'[29] Patterns of violence included physical, verbal, sexual, and financial. Childhood exposure was defined as being within sight or sound of the violence or witnessing the aftermath of the violence (e.g., mother's injuries, property destruction, police intervention to remove the abuser, moving to a domestic violence shelter).[30]

Initial purposive sampling criteria included females who met the following criteria: 1) twenty-one or older, 2) not living in their parents' home/childhood residence, and 3) had experienced (during childhood) their mothers being abused by intimate male partners in the household in which they were reared.

---

27 Li-yu Song and Chaiw-yi Shih, 'Recovery from Partner Abuse: The Application of the Strengths Perspective,' *International Journal of Social Welfare* 19 (2010): 2.

28 Roche and Wood, 'A Narrative Principle for Feminist Social Work with Survivors of Male Violence,' 465–475.

29 Jeffrey L. Edleson et al., 'Assessing Child Exposure to Adult Domestic Violence,' *Children and Youth Services Review* 20 (2007): 963.

30 Howard Meltzer et al., 'The Mental Health of Children who Witness Domestic Violence,' *Child and Family Social Work* 14 (2009): 491–501.

Subsequent theoretical sampling was based on the qualitative criteria of saturation of the code categories, relevance to emerging themes, and added variation of perspective (e.g., diversity in demographics, duration of IPV, etc.).[31] Based on the sampling criteria, of the 35 inquiries received, 26 met sampling criteria, and 15 of those agreed to become research participants and complete in-person interviews.

3.2 *Participant Information*

Participants were women ranging in age from twenty-two to sixty-four-years-old ($M = 39$, $SD = 11$). The majority were European American ($n = 11$), one was Hispanic, one was African American, one was Asian, and one was Native American. Of the fifteen participants, twelve were heterosexual, two identified as a lesbian and one identified as a bisexual. Educationally, six had high school degrees and nine participants had completed a bachelor's and/or master's degrees. Most ($n = 13$) had children of their own.

The majority of study participants ($n = 13$) were exposed to the abuser's violence for thirteen or more years with ten out of fifteen reporting that the violence was present throughout their childhoods. The types of violence reported by all participants included physical and emotional abuse, and ten reported that the batterer used weapons including guns, knives, and/or automobiles. Abusers included fathers ($n = 14$) and one stepfather. Nine of the fifteen participants had directly experienced verbal and physical child abuse from the abuser. Although no participants were in an abusive relationship at the time of the study, eight out of fifteen had previously experienced IPV.

3.3 *Procedure*

Although a semi-structured interview of open-ended questions was used, researchers adopted a number of feminist interviewing techniques.[32] For example, participants determined the emphasis they would place on different aspects of their stories and were given the freedom to describe the meaning they had given to their own experiences. Each interview began by the researchers asking participants to pick a pseudonym and to share their childhood experiences of exposure to their mothers' abuse. Participants were also asked about personal qualities and social conditions in relationship to their recovery

31 Julianne S. Oktay, 'Grounded Theory,' *The Qualitative Research Experience*, ed. D. Padgett (Belmont, CA: Wadsworth/Thomson Learning, 2004), 23–46.

32 Shulamit Reinharz and Lynn Davidman, *Feminist Methods in Social Research* (New York: Oxford University Press, 1992).

process, including schematic changes in how they viewed themselves, their parents, and their abuse exposure. Each in-depth interview was approximately an hour and a half. Member (participant) checking included a 30-minute follow-up interview after participants had received a summary of the findings to gain their insights regarding the final analysis. At the conclusion of the second interview, participants were given a $20.00 gift certificate to a national department store.

3.4 *Data Analysis*

Data analysis was conducted using a constant comparative method; a qualitative procedure that identifies and extracts significant statements or 'meaningful units' from in-depth interview transcripts to be conceptualized and reconstructed in new ways.[33] Data were coded and organized by two researchers using the qualitative data analysis program, ATLAS/ti.[34] Initially, analysis involved searching for units of data (i.e., personal qualities, social conditions) that could stand on their own and were associated with the overall purpose for the study. Through coding, data were then grouped into final categories that represented key psychosocial issues and patterns (i.e., childhood powerlessness, adult empowerment) related to recovery, which were analysed by comparing them with one another, so that relevant themes (i.e., altered cognitive schemas regarding deconstructing, reforming and transcending childhood perceptions) addressing the research questions could emerge. Finally, a conceptual framework of the recovery process was generated around the core category (i.e., transforming childhood powerlessness) that described the central phenomenon relating to participants' experiences.

4 Results

4.1 *The Recovery Process: Transforming Childhood Powerlessness*

The recovery process for these adult daughters included a journey of self-discovery (starting with childhood in a violent home) often characterized by confusion and undeserved guilt, always distinguished by powerlessness, to a state of personal power and the possibility of choice (in adulthood). Three

33 Norman K. Denzin and Yvonna S. Lincoln, *The Landscape of Qualitative Research* (Thousand Oaks, CA: SAGE Publications, 1998).

34 James W. Drisko, 'Qualitative Data Analysis Software: A User's Appraisal,' *The Qualitative Research Experience*, ed. D. Padgett (Belmont, CA: Wadsworth/ Thomson Learning, 2004), 189–209.

progressive, yet not mutually exclusive, stages were germane to transforming childhood powerlessness into adult empowerment: deconstruction of childhood beliefs, reformation of childhood misperceptions, and transcendence of childhood experiences. Although participants' recovery journeys may have varied in months or years, they all experienced each stage in their own time and way. Additionally, each stage did not correspond with years of exposure or age (e.g., years away from residing with parents); instead, progressing in the recovery process was reflective of task accomplishment for each stage rather than the passage of time. Recognition, understanding, and acceptance of the past paved the way for seizing personal power in adulthood; it is the heart of the recovery process presented here.

4.2 *Stage One: Deconstruct Childhood Beliefs*

Participants reported belief in the falsehoods told by their fathers (mother is to blame), feelings of anger toward their mothers (for not protecting or for not leaving), and the sense of guilt and self-blame often experienced by children exposed to violence and the abuse of close others. They reported the importance of recognizing their distorted beliefs by making sense of the actions of the abuser, by placing rightful blame on them for making the choices they did. The process of demystifying the past enabled these adult daughters, with the perspective that time and new knowledge provided, to see more clearly the impetus behind those actions. They reported breaking down old beliefs that the abuse was deserved or motivated by anything other than the need for control.

> I think even then I knew I was just afraid but I didn't really know what I was afraid of and I think it was that I was just afraid of the powers that he had in that situation and now when I look at it, then I didn't know that, but now it is like it was just a big power struggle. (Joanna, age 22)

Many participants reported they placed the blame on their mothers, for not leaving, for "causing" the abuse, for not somehow stopping it from happening. They reported memories of blaming their mothers and sometimes themselves for the abuse, often believing in the distorted picture created by the abuser.

> I kind of made her out to be a monster. My dad bashed her to us a lot. I made her out to be a monster, which is weird because she was the victim. But I think maybe my dad was bashing her a lot, which probably helped me with the whole monster personification of her. I don't see her as a monster anymore at all. (Janie, age 36)

Participants also talked of coming to recognize and appreciate more about why their mothers may have stayed in the relationship, and of the idea that people are defined and confined by their time and place, that everyone simply does the best they can with the resources they have.

> I think too she [mother] just didn't want to admit that it failed or that she couldn't change it. If staying with him meant that we had a father no matter what kind of father he was that seemed like the better option for her. (Joanna, age 22)

In addition to illustrating a newfound understanding of the often absence of choice for those suffering from the abuse, the following quote also points to the confusing position of children exposed to violence perpetrated by a loved one – having to reconcile loving a person while fearing and hating their actions.

> Maybe there was nothing that really, physically, that I could have done. He was a lot bigger than me, stronger than me. Maybe I finally understood what my mom was going through. I didn't at first. Sometimes I feel bad about loving my dad so much. Even after what he did. (Tiffany, age 29)

Education about the dynamics and unacceptability of abuse provided empowering information that allowed participants a new window onto the nature of family relationships and became a lasting vehicle for the construction of life beyond abuse. Having attained a new level of consciousness about family violence, participants looked back with new eyes on what seemed true at the time; they then turned these new eyes toward a different present and better future.

> My father was very skilled at saying to my mother, saying to us, you're not going to be anything, so don't even try. And so, just realizing today, I am something today, whatever it is. Today I'm something. And even when you can't get out of bed, you're something, you know? (Casey, age 40)

4.3 *Stage Two: Reform Childhood Misperceptions*

Once on a path toward a new understanding of the past, the recovery process proposed here continued with reforming childhood misperceptions through replacing distorted beliefs, particularly regarding their parents, with more realistic and comprehensive perspectives. Participants spoke of sorting through the experiences of the past and what was passed to them by each parent, finding and keeping what was useful, while rejecting the rest. This perspective empowered them to sift through experiences and gain valuable knowledge that would enrich their lives in the future.

> I think that he [father] taught us how to keep our guard up and kind of look out for ourselves. I think we were intelligent enough to pull out the good and learn from it. I pulled good out of the aggressive and the loving out of the passive and kind of combined it. I think that is what's so good about the way I was raised is that I realized that you can't just walk away sometimes. You just can't. (Moberly, age 32)

> My dad was very smart. He was a voracious reader, and I am too. My mom was, in spite of everything, pull yourself up by your bootstraps and do. So those things that I took from my parents are good things, and they're things I'm proud of, but I'm leaving the rest of it behind. (Maggie, age 45)

Feelings of self-respect coupled with respect for the fortitude of women and other survivors – most especially their mothers – appeared significant in reforming their perceptions.

> I think she was in an age where she didn't know what to do and so she didn't do anything. She could have left, but I don't think that ever occurred to her. I think she could have protected us, but I think she had more than she could handle to try to protect herself. Looking back, now that she's gone, I think about how she got up every day and went on with her life knowing what was going to happen that day. I just feel sorry for her that she didn't have any more options, you know? And being Catholic of course, God wasn't going to help you either. You didn't even pray for help because that was your lot. You were married forever and that was the way it was going to be and I don't think she had a soul she could talk to. (Susan, age 34)

Several described a more comprehensive understanding of their fathers, and as a result, having empathy for them while not condoning their violent actions.

> I couldn't hate my dad ever and to imagine what kind of pain that he was going through to do that to me and my mom when I knew he loved us very much. (Melissa, age 27)

> I really didn't hold any grudge against my dad, I felt that was just the way he was. I knew how my grandparents had been towards him and probably made him that way and so he was an angry young man. (Susan, age 34)

For some, but certainly not all participants, the act of parental forgiveness served as a path to accept the past and move beyond it.

> You do your best at the time with the information and knowledge that you have. I don't think anybody intentionally makes bad decisions for their kids. I guess I just accept my parents for who they are and try to forgive them I guess. (Diane, age 27)

The following participant's quote reflects her notion of "selfish" forgiveness, not done to exonerate the perpetrator, but rather as a tool for releasing the past from the grip of bitter and unresolved memories – although they may indeed remain unresolved, they can be left behind.

> What else can you do but to forgive him? But if I sit here and tell you I've forgotten, I'm lying. I will never forget. There is no way I can forget. The memory is just too huge and too painful, and I cannot forget. But I do forgive. I guess it's a selfish act, for my sake, I forgive, so I can move on. (Suria, age 35)

As participants came to see both parents more clearly and began to accept those realities, they also found acceptance for themselves. Akin to self-forgiveness, this is meaningful both in the process of acceptance as well as in the ability as adults to write their own lives, and do better than what the past might predict.

> I have to learn, too, to meet myself where I'm at, on any given day. It could be different, you know, depending on what triggers me, or what's going on. (Casey, age 40).

> Everybody is just doing the best they can, so that's all I can do is just do the best I can. And I can't control everything and whatever is going to happen is going to happen. I can either be positive about it and adapt to the changes, or I can continue to be a very rigid black-and-white person. (Maggie, age 45)

The process of reforming childhood misconceptions and accepting the past did not occur in isolation. Each participant noted the influence of spirituality or religion, professional therapeutic intervention or support group involvement, formal education, or life experience such as parenting as associated with the need to find a way to move beyond the difficulties of the past. For some, the simple progression of growing, maturing, and gaining life knowledge served to do so.

> I realized I don't want to be in a relationship like that [her parents]. I don't want to be with someone that drinks and I don't want my kids to experience those types of things, and so I learned a lot of what not to do in parenting. (Diane, age 27)

> It wasn't until my mid-30s that I realized that I don't have to endure shit anymore. As soon as I realize I'm trying to endure it instead of rise above it, then I can do something about it. (Casey, age 40)

4.4 *Stage Three: Transcend Childhood Experiences*

Once on a pathway of accepting the past and their parents, participants were more equipped with knowledge and the motivation to take charge of their lives. For these adult daughters, once they realized their own powerlessness to change the events of the past, this provided the avenue for claiming their power as adults. Recognizing that one has not only the right but the power to self-determination was a significant step in their recovery process.

> I have endeavoured, though it was hard, to make ceaseless efforts to take the events of my life, often painful, sometimes unbearable, and transform them into meaningful experiences. So every time I went through something, it was difficult, but I tried to draw strength from it and learn something from it. I learned who I am and it helped me to mature. It helped me to grow. That's why I'm thankful for the people and events in my life because had it not been for them, I may not have grown the way I've grown. It's kind of strange for me to say that, but it's true. (Suria, age 35)

Along with this idea of acting on one's own behalf, participants spoke of the importance of self-reliance to write their own futures, free from the potentially damaging choices of others. These adult daughters spoke of the importance of controlling their own destinies.

> Between the ages of twelve and fourteen, I made up my mind that I was in control of my own destiny, that I couldn't count on anyone around me to help me, to make things better, to take away the pain, and I did that with absolutely everything. (Donna, age 45)

> You need to go to college and make something of yourself, not for the sake of making something of yourself, but because you can't depend on a man to always take care of you. I wanted a profession where I wouldn't be one man away from welfare. (Janie, age 36)

Beyond applying the lesson of self-sufficiency to their own lives, several participants underscored the value of sharing this lesson with their own children.

> In talking with my daughters, I always told them not to rely on men. You don't need men, is what I tell them. They're great to have and you can love them, but you don't need them to survive. I'm making sure that they know that they don't have to count on anybody but themselves. (Mary, age 47)

The profound and hard-won knowledge of what *not* to be in life appears to be of extraordinary value to the process of creating a different life. Participants emphasized the necessity of defining one's values and firmly applying these to their own lives, especially in terms of family, love relationships and parenting, as well as eliminating negative and dangerous elements from their lives.

> It's only in that manner can you know who you are, because you saw who you aren't. It's like that in life, isn't it? If you know what is bad, then you know what good is. That's what happened. It was kind of hard for me to explain that, but that was a good result that I got out of this. (Suria, age 35)

These adult daughters spoke about protecting themselves emotionally and maintaining control over their environment. Sarah, age 64, reported her right to avoid things that remind her of or cause emotional pain stating, 'I refuse to allow myself to be exposed to anything I don't have to that is about pain. Those are the choices I can make.' Many reported having strong feelings about the presence of substance abuse in their lives, either their own or others.' For instance, as a result of witnessing abuse very often perpetrated within the context of alcohol abuse, participants reported their decision to avoid drinking and drugs.

> My brother and I broke the cycle. We don't drink, we don't smoke, we don't do drugs, we don't abuse. I don't like going to bars, I don't like being around people who drink, I don't like it. I have had enough of it in my childhood. (Moberly, age 32)

Above all, participants' responses indicated no tolerance for abuse, based both on what was witnessed during childhood and from limited adult experiences.

Those who shared that they had experienced violence in their own love relationships asserted that what they already knew from childhood informed their ability to leave abuse behind. They reported that intimate partner violence was not to be tolerated, without exception.

> I will not stay in a violent relationship. I said [to intimate partner], 'you know you make me have flashbacks to my step-dad. I don't want to be around that and I will get rid of you. I will dump you.' You have to establish what you're willing to tolerate. (Janie, age 36)

> I've told him [husband] several times in the early years, if you touch me, you better make sure I'm dead, because I'm coming after you. And I told him that in the earlier part of our relationship. 'Don't ever think you can lay a hand on me, because I won't take it.' (Mary, age 47)

The importance of protecting themselves from violence in adult life – when armed with the ability to make independent choices and to shield themselves from further pain – extended as well to the necessity of also safeguarding their own children from experiencing the same.

> The reason why I left him the second time was because I had children already, and they were witnessing. And I'm not going to subject my children to that. I wanted to break the cycle. They need not go through this. They don't deserve this. (Suria, age 35)

For those who chose to have a relationship with their fathers, the perpetrators of violence against their mothers, they did so on their own non-negotiable terms.

> There was a rule that if I drive 70 miles to see you and you're drunk, I'm driving 70 miles home and you won't see my children. I just flat out told him [father] after I got older, a little braver, if you want to see your grandchildren you won't be drunk when I get here. And if you drink while I'm here, then we're going home, because they will not see what I saw as a child. (Maggie, age 45)

Not only a source of pride, but a blueprint for the future, participants expressed determination for a better life than the one they were given as children.

> You are bigger and you came out better for what happened to you. You can blame them [parents] all day long, but in the end, you've come out

> a better person, because you're still alive. And that supersedes anything else that could have happened. You're still alive, you could have been killed easily, or killed yourself many, many times. (Maggie, age 45)

> But I did not walk that path [of violence]. I fought to stay sane and become better than that. I never did walk the other way, and think, 'I'll just give up on my life. It's just bad as bad can be. Let me just go and be bad too.' It's just easier to walk that way, but I refused. (Suria, age 35)

In summary, recovery involved a process of cognitive deconstruction and reordering of the distortions of childhood toward a state of intentional choice-making and creation of one's own life, according to the drive to leave abuse in the past and to establish a future informed by the lessons of past hardship and pain. Generally not experienced as a moment of epiphany, the path to a new consciousness and better life began with participants' need for closure and the freedom to focus on the future rather than the past.

5 Discussion

The key phenomenon for the participants in the current study was transforming childhood powerlessness into adult empowerment by progressing through the following stages: deconstruction of childhood beliefs, reformation of childhood misperceptions, and transcendence of childhood experiences. In the initial stage it was important for participants to recognize the past, including childhood misconceptions, and to deconstruct these negative beliefs often based on acquired knowledge regarding IPV dynamics. Yet awareness of such issues as power and powerlessness within in a violence context did not end at the initial stage but was accentuated through the process. In the next stage, being informed was put into action as participants replaced childhood beliefs and misperceptions with a more comprehensive understanding of their parents, inclusive of both positive and negative qualities, allowing for an acceptance of the past, while not condoning the violence. In the final stage, participants recognized that their childhood powerlessness was a part of their past, but did not have to be a part of their future. Thus, transcending their childhood experiences included closure of the past while owning one's power in the present to create the identity and life they desired, including a commitment to breaking the cycle of violence.

The common experience of powerlessness shared by mothers and children living with violence in the family emerged as a significant facet of recovery and empowerment in adulthood – what was lost for them as children became a driving force in the creation of a better future. Although none of our participants labelled their experiences of establishing an adult identity as "feminist consciousness-raising" clearly their process embraced feminist ideals and personal empowerment.[35] In coming to see the powerlessness and trap in which their mothers lived, participants also recognized that they too had no way of – and therefore no accountability for – stopping the abuse. The decision by adult daughters to take charge of their own lives, the drive toward self-actualization, and the grasping of personal power served as a well of hope to be drawn upon.

The process of adaptation in the aftermath of a traumatic event appears to involve a recognition and ability to manage uncertainty, one's cognitions and emotions, and recognition of humans as imperfect.[36] Acknowledgment of capacities and limitations within themselves and their parents allowed these adult daughters to gain a beneficial mixture of acceptance for the past and optimism for the future. Participants were able to see that despite the past, the future could be different and that the events of childhood did not destine them to repeat history for the rest of their lives. Consequently, these adult daughters expressed a staunch refusal to not let the past contaminate the future.

Regardless of the route that brought each participant to understand her power to transcend the past, many expressed the value and meaning of this realization. Despite the pain, adult daughters took not only pride but also a unique wisdom with them as they left the past behind. Linley and Joseph present the concept of wisdom as one emerging from life experience that can be understood as both process and outcome.[37] Pride in surviving the past is further understood as finding value in the difficult lessons that many who are fortunate enough to not live in a violent home may not have the benefit of.

6 Implications

For children, both short- and long-term psychological and physical development are impacted by exposure to IPV.[38] Given the prevalence and the

35 Carolyn J. Black, 'Translating Principles into Practice: Implementing the Feminist and Strengths Perspectives in Work with Battered Women,' *Affilia* 18.3 (2003): 332–349.

36 P. Alex Linley and Stephen Joseph, 'Positive Change Following Trauma and Adversity: A Review,' *Journal of Traumatic Stress* 17.1 (2004): 11–21.

37 Ibid.

38 Robert A. Geffner, Robyn S. Igelman and Jennifer Zellner, 'Introduction: Children Exposed to Interpersonal Violence: A Need for Additional Research and Validated Treatment Programs,' *Journal of Emotional Abuse* 3.1 (2003): 1–10.

likelihood of encountering adult daughters, who during childhood were exposed to IPV, mental health and health professionals should screen for such experiences in assessing their clients' current functioning. More must be done to reach out to adult daughters of abuse survivors to speed their recovery and help them regain their personal sense of power and agency. Under the assertion that cognitive schemas are altered by traumatic exposure, Constructivist Self-Development Theory (CDST) frames intervention as aiming to repair or replace problematic schema that may contribute to risk-taking, poor decision-making, and disrupted well-being. Therefore, altering childhood beliefs and schemas about violence can fundamentally affect how childhood exposure becomes manifested for daughters in their own adult lives.

This study's findings offer enhanced knowledge of recovery for adult daughters and provide the following conceptual framework for helping professionals and survivors seeking signposts on the journey toward healing.

1. *Deconstruct childhood beliefs*. Deconstructing one's assumptions and worldview in the aftermath of trauma appears to be a precursor to a cognitive re-ordering of new and experience-informed ideas for adult daughters. Recognition of distorted thinking and misunderstandings during childhood, particularly about the nature of the perpetrator's violence, is a crucial step toward the creation of a life free of violence.
2. *Reform childhood misperceptions*. Equipping adult daughters with knowledge and the motivation to realize the possibility of life without abuse, they may take steps toward fully accepting and making meaning of the events of childhood as the foundation for their future. Acceptance of both the shortcomings and the acts of personal power demonstrated by parents is important not only to realize the true dynamics of the situation, but also for the process of allowing oneself the room to move forward with tools and information that were absent in the past. This re-forming of impacted cognitive schemas allows adults to move forward with a new lens with which to view the self and others.
3. *Transcend childhood experiences*. With acceptance of the past and the grasping of one's own power to choose a different path, adult daughters may be assisted toward creating for themselves a new context in which to create a different life course (than their parents). By accepting both one's own limitations and also one's power and desire for a better life, adult daughters may work toward closure of the past while generating a divergent future, paved by their own choices and illuminated by their hard-earned lessons of life.

A feminist practice approach combined with cognitive therapy or a narrative/deconstructive strategy are suggested by the findings here as helpful tools to assist in the recovery process. Although individual counselling can be effective,

Roche and Wood make a convincing argument for the power of group work to enhance individual transformation by embracing collective empowerment.[39] Groups specifically for adult daughters focused on helping women understand the dynamics of abuse that impacted their mothers, may be powerful forces for positive intergenerational change.

The goal of the helping process should not be for helping professionals to impose a recovery framework onto survivors' life experiences. However, we should not preclude ourselves from having these types of conversation with clients, as practitioners can find ways to support this process of growth, even if they cannot create it. Further research is necessary in this emerging area in order to advance theory and to develop conceptual models regarding recovery for this population.

7 Limitations of Study

The purposive sample for this exploratory study came from and around a small Midwestern city in the United States. It is possible that the experiences of urban adult daughters may be shaped differently by the inherent differences between rural and urban settings. This exploratory study was based on a small sample size with limited ethnic and racial diversity and included the possibility of selection bias with regard to the decision to participate in the study. Participants in this sample were also well educated and there may be different pathways to recovery based on level of education. Finally, data collected through in-depth interviews rely on the self-reported memories of people who have experienced trauma. It is not uncommon for people who have experienced trauma to minimize their experiences as a way of coping.[40]

8 Conclusion

Although feminist helping strategies are available to assist women in transforming their lives to overcome male violence,[41] information is lacking

39 Roche and Wood, 'A Narrative Principle for Feminist Social Work with Survivors of Male Violence,' 465–475.

40 Guy Enoch and Eli Buchbinder, 'The Interactive Construction of Narrative Styles in Sensitive Interviews: The Case of Domestic Violence Research,' *Qualitative Inquiry* 11 (2005): 588–617.

41 Roche and Wood, 'A Narrative Principle for Feminist Social Work with Survivors of Male Violence,' 465–475.

regarding the recovery process for individuals who during childhood witnessed their mothers being abused.[42] For these adult daughters, their process involved deconstructing childhood beliefs, righting childhood misperceptions, and transcending their childhood adversity, based on self-beliefs of choice and self-determination. This is the essence of empowerment and was significant in their recovery process. Although abuse may seem to consume, it cannot erase the individual inside, nor the ability to survive and become something beautiful, despite the ugliness of the past.

Bibliography

Aldwin, Carolyn M. and Michael R. Levenson. 'Posttraumatic Growth: Developmental Perspective.' *Psychological Inquiry* 15.1 (2004): 19–22.

Anderson, Kim M. and Eun-Jun Bang. 'Assessing PTSD and Resilience for Females who during Childhood were Exposed to Domestic Violence.' *Child & Family Social Work* 17.1 (2012): 55–65.

Anderson, Kim, Fran Danis and Kirsten Havig. 'Adult daughters of battered women: Recovery and posttraumatic growth following childhood adversity.' *Families in Society: The Journal of Contemporary Social Services* 92.2 (2011): 154–160.

Artz, Sibelle, Margaret A. Jackson, Katherine R. Rossiter, Alicia Nijdam-Jones, István Géczy and Sheila Porteous. 'A Comprehensive Review of the Literature on the Impact of Exposure to Intimate Partner Violence on Children and Youth.' *Journal of Child, Youth and Family Studies* 5.4 (2014): 493–587.

Bair-Merritt, Megan, Barry Zuckerman, Marilyn Augustyn and Peter F. Cronholm. 'Silent victims – An Epidemic of Childhood Exposure to Domestic Violence.' *The New England Journal of Medicine* 369.18 (2013): 1673–1675

Becker, Kimberly D., Jeffrey Stuewig and Laura A. McClosky. 'Traumatic Stress Symptoms of Women Exposed to Different Forms of Childhood Victimization and Intimate Partner Violence.' *Journal of Interpersonal Violence* 25.9 (2010): 1699–1715.

Black, Carolyn J. 'Translating Principles into Practice: Implementing the Feminist and Strengths Perspectives in Work with Battered Women.' *Affilia* 18.3 (2003): 332–349.

42 Kim Anderson, Fran Danis, and Kirsten Havig, 'Adult Daughters of Battered Women: Recovery and Posttraumatic Growth Following Childhood Adversity,' *Families in Society: The Journal of Contemporary Social Services* 92. 2 (2011): 154–160; Janice C. Humphreys, 'Turnings and Adaptations in Resilient Daughters of Battered Women,' *Journal of Nursing Scholarship* 33.3 (2001): 245–251.

Burke, Nadine J., Julia L. Hellman, Brandon G. Scott, Carl F. Weems and Victor G. Carrion. 'The Impact of Adverse Childhood Experiences on an Urban Pediatric Population.' *Child Abuse and Neglect* 35 (2011): 408–413.

Calhoun, Lawrence G. and Richard G. Tedeschi. 'Beyond Recovery from Trauma: Implications for Clinical Practice and Research.' *Journal of Social Issues* 54.2 (1998): 357–371.

Cater, Asa K., Laura E. Miller, Kathryn H. Howell, and Sandra A. Graham-Bermann. 'Childhood Exposure to Intimate Partner Violence and Adult Mental Health Problems: Relationships with Gender and Age of Exposure.' *Journal of Family Violence* 30 (2015): 875–886.

Chartier, Mariette, John R. Walker and Barbara Naimark. 'Seperate and Cumulative Effects of Adverse Childhood Experiences in Predicting Adult Health and Health Care Utilization.' *Child Abuse and Neglect* 34 (2010): 454–464.

Clements, Caroline M., Claire Oxtoby and Richard L. Ogle. 'Methodological Issues in Assessing Psychological Adjustment in Child Witnesses of Intimate Partner Violence.' *Trauma, Violence and Abuse* 9.2 (2008): 114–127.

Davies, Corrie A., David DiLillo and Isaac G. Martinez. 'Isolating Adult Psychological Correlates of Witnessing Parental Violence: Findings from a Predominantly Latina Sample.' *Journal of Family Violence* 19.6 (2004): 377–385.

Denzin, Norman K. and Yvonna S. Lincoln. *The Landscape of Qualitative Research.* Thousand Oaks, CA: SAGE Publications, 1998.

Drisko, James W. 'Qualitative Data Analysis Software: A User's Appraisal.' *The Qualitative Research Experience*, edited by D. Padgett, 189–209. Belmont, CA: Wadsworth/ Thomson Learning, 2004.

Dube, Shanta R., Robert F. Anda, Vincent J. Felitti, Valerie J. Edwards and David F. Williamson. 'Exposure to Abuse, Neglect, and Household Dysfunction among Adults who Witnessed Intimate Partner Violence as Children: Implications for Health and Social Services.' *Violence and Victims* 17.1 (2002): 3–17.

Edleson, Jeffrey L., Amanda L. Ellerton, Ellen A. Seagren, Staci L. Kirchberg, Sarah O. Schmidt and Amirthini T. Ambrose. 'Assessing Child Exposure to Adult Domestic Violence.' *Children and Youth Services Review* 20 (2007): 961–971.

Edwards, Valerie J., Robert F. Anda, Vincent J. Felitti, and Shanta R. Dube. 'Adverse Childhood Experiences and Health-Related Quality of Life as an Adult.' *Health Consequences of Abuse in the Family: A Clinical Guide for Evidence-Based Practice*, edited by K. A. Kendall-Tackett, 81–94. Washington, DC: American Psychological Association, 2004.

Enoch, Guy and Eli Buchbinder. 'The Interactive Construction of Narrative Styles in Sensitive Interviews: The Case of Domestic Violence Research.' *Qualitative Inquiry* 11 (2005): 588–617.

Evans, Sarah, Corrie Davies and David DiLillo. 'Exposure to Domestic Violence: A Meta-Analysis of Child and Adolescent Outcomes.' *Aggression & Violent Behaviour* 13.2 (2008): 131–140.

Fagan, Abigail A. and Emily M. Wright. 'Gender Differences in the Effects of Exposure to Intimate Partner Violence on Adolescent Violence and Drug Use.' *Child Abuse and Neglect* 35.7 (2011): 543–550.

Felitti, Vincent J., Robert F. Anda, Dale Nordenberg, David F. Williamson, Allison M. Spitz, Valerie J. Edwards, Mary P. Koss and James S. Marks. 'Relationship of Childhood Abuse and Household Dysfunction to Many of the Leading Causes of Death in Adults: The Adverse Childhood Experiences (ACE) Study.' *American Journal of Preventive Medicine* 14.4 (1998): 245–258.

Geffner, Robert A., Robyn S. Igelman and Jennifer Zellner. 'Children Exposed to Interpersonal Violence: A Need for Additional Research and Validated Treatment Programs.' *Journal of Emotional Abuse* 3.1/2 (2003): 1–10.

Herrera, Veronica M. and Laura A. McCloskey. 'Gender Differences in the Risk for Delinquency among Youth Exposed to Family Violence.' *Child Abuse and Neglect* 25 (2001): 1037–1051.

Holt, Stephanie, Helen Buckley and Sadhbh Whelan. 'The Impact of Exposure to Domestic Violence on Children and Young People: A Review of the Literature.' *Child Abuse and Neglect* 32 (2008): 797–810.

Holt, Jessica and Wayne Gillespie. 'Intergenerational Transmission of Violence, Threatened Egoism, and Reciprocity: A Test of Multiple Psychosocial Factors Affecting Intimate Partner Violence.' *American Journal of Criminal Justice* 33.2 (2008): 252–266.

Howell, Kathryn H. and Laura E. Miller-Graff. 'Protective Factors Associated with Resilient Functioning in Young Adulthood after Childhood Exposure to Violence.' *Child Abuse and Neglect* 38.12 (2014): 1985–1994.

Humphreys, Janice C. 'Turnings and Adaptations in Resilient Daughters of Battered Women.' *Journal of Nursing Scholarship* 33.3 (2001): 245–251.

Ireland, Timothy O. and Caroline Smith. 'Living in Partner-Violent Families: Developmental Links to Antisocial Behaviour and Relationship Violence.' *Journal of Youth and Adolescence* 38 (2009): 323–339.

Jenney, Angelique, Ramona Allagia and Mark Niepage. 'The lie is that it's not going to get better: Narratives of resilience from childhood exposure to Intimate Partner Violence.' *International Journal of Child and Adolescent Resilience* 4.1 (2016): 64–76.

Kitzmann, Katherine M., Noni K. Gaylord, Aimee R. Holt and Erin D. Kenny. 'Child Witnesses to Domestic Violence: A Meta-Analytic Review.' *Journal of Consulting and Clinical Psychology* 71 (2003): 339–352.

Lamers-Winkelman, Francien, Agnes M. Willeman and Margreet Visser. 'Adverse Childhood Experiences of Referred Children Exposed to Intimate Partner Violence: Consequences for Their Wellbeing.' *Child Abuse and Neglect* 36 (2012): 166–179.

Linley, P. Alex and Stephen Joseph. 'Positive Change Following Trauma and Adversity: A Review.' *Journal of Traumatic Stress* 17.1 (2004): 11–21.

Maker, Azmaira H., Markus Kemmelmeier and Christopher Peterson. 'Long-Term Psychological Consequences in Women of Witnessing Parental Physical Conflict and Experiencing Abuse in Childhood.' *Journal of Interpersonal Violence* 13.5 (1998): 574–589.

Margolin, Gayla and Katrina A. Vickerman. 'Post-Traumatic Stress in Children and Adolescents Exposed to Family Violence: Overview and Issues.' *Couple and Family Psychology: Research and Practice* 1 (2011): 63–73.

Meltzer, Howard, Lucy Doos, Panos Vostanis, Tamsin Ford and Robert Goodman. 'The Mental Health of Children who Witness Domestic Violence.' *Child and Family Social Work* 14 (2009): 491–501.

McDonald Renee, Ernest N. Jouriles, Suhasini Ramisetty-Mikler, Raul Caetano and Charles E. Green. 'Estimating the Number of American Children Living in Partner-Violent Families.' *Journal of Family Psychology* 20.1 (2006): 137–142.

McFarlane, Judith M., Janet Y. Groff, Jennifer A. O'Brien and Kathy Watson. 'Behaviors of Children who are Exposed and Not Exposed to Intimate Partner Violence: An Analysis of 330 Black, White, and Hispanic Children.' *Pediatrics* 112 (2003): e202–e207.

McLaughlin, Katie A., Laura D. Kubzansky, Erin C. Dunn, Robert Waldinger, George Vaillant, and Karestan C. Koenen. 'Childhood Social Environment, Emotional Reactivity to Stress, and Mood and Anxiety Disorders across the Life Course.' *Depression and Anxiety* 27 (2010): 1087–1094.

Moon, Michelle. 'Retrospective Reports of Interparental Abuse by Adult Children from Intact Families.' *Journal of Interpersonal Violence* 15 (2000): 1323–1331.

Onyskiw, Judee E. 'Domestic Violence and Children's Adjustment: A Review of Research.' *Journal of Emotional Abuse* 3 (2003): 11–45.

Oktay, Julianne S. 'Grounded Theory.' *The Qualitative Research Experience*, edited by D. Padgett, 23–46. Belmont, CA: Wadsworth/Thomson Learning, 2004.

Ponce, Allison N., Michelle K. Williams, and George J. Allen. 'Experience of Maltreatment as a Child and Acceptance of Violence in Adult Intimate Relationships: Mediating Effects of Distortions in Cognitive Schemas.' *Violence and Victims* 19.1 (2004): 97–108.

Reinharz, Shulamit and Lynn Davidman. *Feminist Methods in Social Research*. New York: Oxford University Press, 1992.

Reynolds, Mathew W., Joanna Wallace, Tyra F. Hill, Mark D. Weist and Laura A. Nabors. 'The Relationship between Gender, Depression, and Self-Esteem in Children who have Witnessed Domestic Violence.' *Child Abuse and Neglect* 25 (2001): 1201–1206.

Roche, Susan E. and Gayle G. Wood. 'A Narrative Principle for Feminist Social Work with Survivors of Male Violence.' *Affilia* 20.4 (2005): 465–475.

Russell, David, Kristen W. Springer, and Emily A. Greenfield. 'Witnessing Domestic Abuse in Childhood as an Independent Risk Factor for Depressive Symptoms in Adulthood.' *Child Abuse and Neglect* 34 (2010): 448–453.

Saakvitne, Karen W., Howard Tennen, and Glen Affleck. 'Exploring Thriving in the Context of Clinical Trauma Theory: Constructivist Self Development Theory.' *Journal of Social Issues* 54.2 (1998): 279–299.

Song, Li-Yu and Chaiw-Yi Shih. 'Recovery from Partner Abuse: The Application of the Strengths Perspective.' *International Journal of Social Welfare* 19 (2010): 23–32.

Suzuki, Staci L., Robert Geffner and Steven F. Bucky. 'The Experiences of Adults Exposed to Intimate Partner Violence as Children: An Exploratory Qualitative Study of Resilience and Protective Factors.' *Journal of Emotional Abuse* 8.1/2 (2008): 103–121.

CHAPTER 2

Living with Someone both Here and Gone: Trauma and Dementia

Catherine Ann Collins

Abstract

Globally, the World Health Organization estimates that more than 35 million people are living with dementia; that number will triple by 2050, making it a public health priority. As a progressive syndrome, dementia stresses the care recipient in insidious ways, but family and caregivers are also seriously impacted: formally in their role relationship with the parent or spouse, and physically and psychologically because of the emotional stress of caring for someone with Alzheimer's or other forms of dementia. Pauline Boss argues that 'dementia creates ambiguous loss,' a loss for which 'there is no possibility of closure'[1] because the loss of the person you knew, and the relationship you had, comes and goes from moment to moment. For some caregivers the ambiguity and pre-death grief leads to post-traumatic stress. Since living with dementia prevents closure, this chapter turns to strategies for coping with the trauma of dementia. Three concepts coming out of the wrap-up session at the TTP 3 conference have special relevance to this project: (1) how ambiguity exacerbates the trauma for patient and family, (2) the role of repetition in manifestations of the disease and the stress felt by family and caregivers, and (3) how telling stories restores agency and thereby provides a way of responding to the trauma of dementia. Because storytelling bears witness to recovery from trauma and the narratives demystify the ambiguous loss of coping with dementia, I have included stories as a central mode of expression in this chapter.

Keywords

ambiguity – ambiguous loss – closure – dementia – repetition – storytelling – trauma

•••

1 Pauline Boss, 'The Trauma and Complicated Grief of Ambiguous Loss,' *Pastoral Psychology* 59 (2010): 137.

 | DOI:10.1163/9789004397576_004

The Day We Figured It Out
The phone rang as I was on my way to class. Mom needed me to come to their house right away and take Dad to the doctor's clinic; he was really sick. They had told her that if I got him out there right away he could be seen. When we arrived the receptionist said no doctors were on duty; that she had clearly told my mother to take him to the Emergency Room. I thought it odd that a retired RN would hear a medical issue so incorrectly, but we rushed to the hospital. Dad stayed there: I took Mom home and promised to take her to see him in the morning. When I picked her up the next day she was frustrated, almost angry. She told me Dad had been outside all night and she called and called for him to come in and go to bed, but he didn't come in. "But when you walked in I remembered he was in the hospital, not outside all night. I guess I just forgot." Dad died 5 days later. I never took her back to her home; something was really wrong. She lived with me for 6 weeks and then moved into an independent living unit – the care coordinators said her memory issues were not severe enough to warrant Assisted Living. My brothers and I agreed. We were all wrong.[2]

1 Introduction

John Berger argues, 'Memory implies a certain act of redemption. What is remembered has been saved from nothingness. What is forgotten is abandoned.'[3] Although Berger is writing about photography, the comment struck me as singularly apt in explaining why dementia is traumatic for those who watch it happen, name their loved one as having the disease, and explore their own anger, frustration, and eventually acceptance of what it feels like to experience being forgotten. Relationships are, after all, partially created, valued, and even judged by shared memories in the form of casual conversations, predictable role-governed behaviours, and family stories that are told. These modes

2 Some of the stories that I have included, like this one, are my own. Others have been borrowed from friends who told them to me when I needed to gain perspective on Mom's dementia, and later sent them to me for inclusion in this chapter.

3 John Berger, *About Looking* (New York: Vintage International, 1980), 58.

of communication enact shared moments of redemption that constitute us as a family unit. Yet the interactions themselves traumatize patient and family members alike when conversations become impossible because memories are gone or the words do not come out, when the parent becomes the child in his or her behaviours or dependency, when the child must make even the little decisions for the parent – what to order at the restaurant, when to go to the bathroom, what is permissible vocalized observation in public situations – and when the important moments that are ritually retold at family gatherings are all new and often insignificant to the one living with dementia. Ambiguity about what is appropriate to say or do replaces comfortable predictability because memory disruptions wipe away the past for the person with dementia, even erasing some members from the family.

> *Rationalizing Forgetfulness Becomes Harder and Harder*
> Mother always flew up for my birthday on October 5th. That year she arrived and never mentioned it. But she was due to fly out that day and said we should go to lunch at the airport. I thought she had something planned. There was no mention of my birthday. One month later, on November 5, I received a card. I had a cousin with the same first and last name that I had before marriage. It was her birthday.

> *And Then We Take It Personally*
> Mother had minor work done on her watch when she visited the year before and the jeweller here didn't charge her. In the intervening year, it had stopped running. The jeweller wanted $60 to work on it. Mother was appalled. So I packaged it up and put it in a side pocket of her carry-on and she flew home. I called to make sure she got home safely. She was very angry with me. She couldn't find her watch and accused me of stealing it. It was a watch I had given her.

I promised myself at the third Trauma Theory and Practice conference that I would try to write about the relationship between dementia and trauma. At the wrap-up session to that conference we talked about the concepts we had collectively explored, focusing on what needed more attention. My notes said we should dig deeper into issues of remembering and forgetting, identity disruption, ways of healing, and ways of experiencing. I listened to a number of papers that reiterated a concern I had explored with respect to trauma – the role of repetition in prolonging trauma. That third trauma conference was also the first time my mother, who suffers from severe dementia, did not have me visiting every other day, and because we had just moved her from an independent living facility to a group home, I knew the changes in her routine would be stressful. I felt guilty for leaving her, especially when my brothers made it clear they had plans that precluded a visit. While I listened and participated in the conference, I concluded that trauma was an apt way to describe dementia's effect on an individual and on the family of someone living with it.

I am not a trained therapist and I do not do research in clinical areas. This chapter therefore is not a traditional analytic chapter – what I am comfortably used to writing. It is instead a narrative of the stories I have told and heard from a set of close friends and colleagues, who like me, have experienced a parent with dementia and the personal trauma inherent in coping with the ambiguity and inexorable progression of the disease in a loved one. Stories are central to who we are as individuals and members of collectives, and this particular collection of stories, and the ruminations that emanate from them, reflect my efforts to make sense of dementia and the trauma it evokes repeatedly, painfully, and unpredictably.

2 Dementia: the Disease

Globally, the World Health Organization estimates that more than 35 million people are living with dementia; that number will triple by 2050, making it a public health priority. As a progressive syndrome, dementia stresses the care recipient in insidious ways, but family caregivers are also seriously impacted: formally in their role relationship with the parent or spouse; and physically and psychologically because of the emotional stress of caring for someone with dementia.

Academic, especially medical literature in the twentieth century, marks senility along with hysteria as 'disorders of memory,'[4] but whether dementia/senility is perceived as a general symptom of old age or a particular medical focus has varied over the decades. Lawrence Cohen notes that with an aging population, Alzheimer's currently is most often discussed as an 'insidious disease' and has opened up discussion of dementia to concerns about ethics and life choices.[5]

Dementia remains a disease that is difficult to diagnose in its early stages, in part because the memory problems seem to come and go, and partially because spouses are frequently complicit in covering for the person living with dementia. Over time, covering dementia's symptoms becomes more difficult. As the

4 Lawrence Cohen, 'Introduction: Thinking about Dementia,' *Thinking about Dementia: Culture, Loss, and the Anthropology of Senility*, ed. Annette Leibing and Lawrence Cohen (New Brunswick, NJ: Rutgers University Press, 2006), 5.

5 Ibid., 8.

disease progresses with symptoms that manifest themselves unpredictably, family and friends find it challenging to predict the interactions they will have with someone with dementia. For example, I talked with a former neighbour who told me the last time she visited Mom she had been surprised that after an absence of six months mother knew her by her full name. Five minutes later her neighbour referred to my youngest brother who has been friends with her son since they were in primary school, but Mom said she didn't know anyone named Rob. Disconcerted by this lapse, Mom's neighbour told me she had quickly said her goodbyes and left, not knowing how to deal with the inconsistency in Mom's ability to remember. Had they gone back to her room she would have pointed out his picture and talked all about him, priding herself in knowing everyone in the photographs. Temporal spatial distortions in this form of dementia make ordinary conversations difficult. Pauline Boss gives a name to what friends and family experience when talking with someone with severe dementia: she argues that 'dementia creates ambiguous loss,' a loss for which there is 'no possibility of closure;'[6] the loss of the person you knew, and the relationship you had, comes and goes from moment to moment. This form of ambiguous loss occurs when the person is physically present but absent psychologically. Boss argues this form of loss is traumatic 'because it is painful, immobilizing, and incomprehensible so that coping is blocked' and may remain so for years; 'the process of bereavement is blocked by an external situation beyond the control of the sufferers.'[7]

Dementia like other traumatic events prevents closure, but I want to explore a strategy for coping that I have learned from my friends who have lived through the ambiguous loss of a family member challenged by the disease. To cope, we have all turned to storytelling, to recounting the remembered moments and the life lessons they teach us. I think it is important to draw a distinction others have made between reminiscing and storytelling. Our stories are intentionally instructive; reminiscences need not be. Incidents are developed into plotlines that allow us to explore the character of our loved one and our own ability/inability to respond to the ambiguous new relationship that the disease seems to thrust upon us when we least expect a change. The lesson often begins with the question: What should I have said or done? Did we wait too long to change her care situation? Is she safe where she is? What can I do to make this less stressful?

Some of what I share here are my own stories, now ready to tell others who are just beginning the process of living with a family member simultaneously

---

6 Boss, 'The Trauma,' 137.

7 Ibid., 140.

here and gone; some are the stories friends told me to help me both laugh and cry when I was once again lulled into thinking things would be stable for a while, that I had a moment to catch my breath and catch up on all those life things that had been postponed to deal with mom's latest crisis.

In telling this story I want to ruminate on repetition as a stressor, and then think about how ambiguity exacerbates the trauma for patient and family, and finally how telling stories restores agency and bears witness to recovery because stories demystify the ambiguous loss of dementia. I approach repetition, ambiguity and storytelling from the perspective of a narrative theorist informed by the theoretical assumptions laid out by Walter Fisher in rhetorical theory,[8] Gerard Genette in literary criticism,[9] and Stanley Hauerwas in religion and ethical studies.[10]

3 Repetition as a Stressor

As a rhetorician I've always regarded repetition as a powerful tool for gaining and sustaining an audience's attention. If, as Kenneth Burke tells us, form is a way of arousing and then fulfilling desires,[11] then

> [*r*]*epetitive form* is the consistent maintaining of a principle under new guises. It is restatement of the same thing in different ways. ... Repetitive form ... is basic to any work of art, or to any other kind of orientation, for that matter. It is our only method of 'talking on the subject.'[12]

Repetition in this sense gives beauty and significance to the message being communicated. Rather than an annoyance, repetition fully engages the audience. But for the person with dementia, repetition is a sign of the disruption of the normal experience of time and context. Repetition distracts, jars the normal flow of conversation, and becomes a sign of the *problem* the dementia patient displays when interacting with others. If it has not happened to you

8 Walter R. Fisher, *Human Communication as Narration: Toward a Philosophy of Reason, Value, and Action* (Columbia SC: University of South Carolina Press, 1987).

9 Gérard Genette, *Narrative Discourse: An Essay in Method*, trans. Jane E. Lewin (Ithaca, New York: Cornell University Press, 1972).

10 Stanley Hauerwas, *A Community of Character: Towards a Constructive Christian Social Ethic* (Notre Dame, IN: University of Notre Dame Press, 1981).

11 Kenneth Burke, *Counter-Statement* (Berkeley, CA: University of California Press, 1968), 124.

12 Ibid., 125.

yet, it will, that moment when you are in the middle of telling a story and you wonder if you've already told it to this group. All of us have momentary memory losses as we age, but this is something more. It reminds me of Unc's *It's a Good Story.*

> *It's A Good Story! They Can Hear It Again*
> Unc was always a storyteller – recounting his fishing trips, or going further back to tell tales of things he had done with my dad when they were boys. In his later years, as the dementia developed, he would tell us the same stories repeatedly whenever he came to visit. When Hazel would remonstrate that we had heard that story before, Unc would always say – "It's a good story! They can hear it again."

It may be a good story, but the repetitive telling, especially the inability to stop sharing the story, signals more than a momentary lapse. Repeated stories become too much when the repetition becomes obsessive, and usually centres on things the dementia patient cannot control. This form of repetition neither creates nor gratifies desire; it resembles Caruth's definition of trauma, a 'wound of the mind' wherein 'the breach of the mind's experience of time, self and the world … is not, like the wound of the body, a simple and healable event.'[13] In these cases, trauma haunts the person; 'the event is not assimilated or experienced fully at the time but only belatedly, in its repeated *possession* of the one who experiences it.'[14] Simple things – a television program, a photograph or smell – can trigger the compulsive repetition, the inability to recall and process the past. When the dementia patient cannot recall the lost memory they repeatedly ask for answers. Unfortunately, rational answers do not seem to satisfy the obsessive need to call up the memory, because it is their inability to retrieve a memory and not your explanation that they desperately need to control in order to break the obsessive cycle. While manifestations of these memory-disruptions signal trauma for the patient they also create stress for family members. Seemingly reasonable conversations suddenly fall apart. The person you thought you were talking to gets caught up in obsessive repetition of fears they are experiencing, and rational reassurances do little to relieve their distress.

> *Was I Married to Your Father?*
> Me: Mom, how are you doing today?

13 Cathy Caruth, *Trauma: Explorations in Memory* (Baltimore: Johns Hopkins University Press, 1995), 4.

14 Ibid., 4–5.

Mom: Well I'm worried. ... Were your dad and I ever married?
Me: Yes Mom, you and Dad were married for almost 65 years.
Mom: Are you sure? I don't think we were.
Me: Mom, you don't need to worry. I have your wedding pictures.
Mom: I think we just told you we were married but we never were.
Me: Mom, your granddaughter Kristin tried on your wedding dress when she was 16, right in your bedroom. You were married. You and Dad and Anna Lee and Joe had the same anniversary. You went out together every year on your anniversary for almost fifty years.
Mom: Are you sure we were married?
Me: Yes mom. Have you been watching television?
Mom: Yes, and the man and woman weren't actually married. When they died the children found out that their parents had never married. I don't think your dad and I were ever married and I don't want my children to find out.
Me: Don't worry Mom, the boys and I know you were married. I even have the marriage certificate in the safe deposit box.
Mom: I'm mad at your brother. You tell Jim to bring Dad back from the cabin. I need him here.
Me: Mom, Dad died almost two years ago.
Mom: He did? Oh, that's right. Did I go to the funeral?
Me: Yes Mom you went to the funeral and we have been to the cemetery to visit and leave flowers.
Mom: I have to ask you something. Do you think your Dad and I were ever married?
Me: Mom, don't worry you and Dad were married. You were watching a TV show where the man and woman weren't married, but you and Dad were married for almost 65 years and I have your wedding pictures. Don't worry.
Mom: Where is your Dad? I'm going to tell him that we need to get married.
Me: Mom, it's time for your dinner now. I'll come back and see you tomorrow. Love you.

I need to remember as I talk with my mother that I am not the argumentation teacher. I need to remember that evidence and reasoning will not allay her fears. Rational explanations are not the answer. Holding her hand, getting her to laugh are better options. The problem emerges from the unpredictability of our interactions these days. For a while the old Mom is there and normal conversation ensues, then without warning she is in another place that I do not understand and from which it is increasing difficult to draw her away. Any repetition on her part triggers stress for all of us. Two days ago my brother's family was in town and visited Mom. It was a bad day. My nephew told me he dreaded the lucid moments the most because then he did not know how to talk to her. When she was in her own world he could just go along with the performance with the complicated explication of her compulsive repetitions. For the person living with dementia repetition becomes a symptom of the disease and an indicator of stress. For family and friends that same repetition becomes the stressor, signalling the unlikelihood of continued conversation.

4 The Ambiguity of Old Identities

She seemed to be fine for days: then she would tell me she had spent the whole night taking care of her patients. The caregiver told me she making rounds, going into other people's rooms, checking to make sure they were in bed, locking their doors. She thought she was still an RN at Salem Hospital and this was her night shift duty. One day I discovered that for at least three days she had not taken the Prednizone she was on. When a nurse cannot manage her meds it is more than old age and minor forgetfulness. I finally got her in to see a cognitive neurologist who, after four other doctors had failed to diagnose anything more than old age, told us Mom had severe temporal and spatial dementia. The doctor asked her why she 'made rounds' each night. She started to answer with the familiar narrative of being a nurse and checking her patients each night. He stopped her midway through this story and asked her if she knew she was no longer a nurse. She thought about his question and said yes, she knew she was retired and living in an apartment but almost immediately returned to the comforting story of being a nurse making rounds of patients who needed her. The story and behaviour comforted her in an old and important identity. If she was a working nurse she need not deal with being institutionalized. In her clearer moments Mom shared her fear – having been raised in an institution (orphanage) she forcefully asserted she wasn't going to die in one. She was aware enough to know there was nothing independent in *independent living* when someone told you when to eat and where to sit and when to go to bed. She was not happy with the loss of control that independent living imposed on her. All she needed to be happy, she told the cognitive neurologist, was to go back to her home and live with her children and husband. Somehow she seemed to know that wasn't possible, so acting out her old identity – head nurse – gave her a purpose, or as McLean explains, telling that life story 'creates a sense of order out of potential meaninglessness.'[15] Her identities as wife, mother, and active volunteer in her church had all changed dramatically in a matter of weeks. Holding on to her old work identity helped her cope with her institutionalization.

Mother has dementia. She can hold onto reality for brief moments, but as soon as she is stressed her conversations have only a subjective coherence for her; they lack coherence for family, friends, and caregivers. Naming her condition helped resolve some of the ambiguity for us. There was no cure, things were not going to get better, but we knew what it was with which she and we would have to learn to live. What we didn't know until much later was how typical her behaviour is for someone with dementia. We also did not realize that time would not make us better decision-makers, but we would find strategies for coping with the ambiguity of Mom's identity. Nursing was an important part of Mom's identity. Although telling us she was still serving aptly in that old role identity had no truth, no current facticity, Peter Coleman argues that importantly, her story could allow us to make sense of her behaviour. It reflects her subjective truth. Scholars exploring life stories and narrative coherence contend that we need to switch our perspective from seeking coherence within an objective narrative of her life to a coherence that inheres with the person's life experiences – that the story must have 'a subjective truth' as understood by the narrator, not one 'determined by an objective observer.'[16] Unfortunately, no doctor helped us to see this. It was in our own storytelling, and in reading academic essays addressing dementia and storytelling that we could, in hindsight, come to understand what she was doing and how it must have made sense to her.

There is a temptation to see in Coleman's take on dementia and narrative coherence relief from the fear that patients experiencing dementia are suffering. If there is a subjective coherence, maybe the flights from reality are not all that painful to the subject. Catherine Malabou's work on the new wounded (those suffering from brain disorders such as her grandmother's Alzheimer's disease) challenges that hope. She theorizes that dementia patients experience brain suffering, and asks:

15 Athena Helen McLean, 'Coherence without Facticity in Dementia: The Case of Mrs. Fine,' *Thinking about Dementia: Culture, Loss, and the Anthropology of Senility*, ed. Annette Leibing and Lawrence Cohen (New Brunswick, NJ: Rutgers University Press, 2006), 172.

16 Peter G. Coleman, 'Creating a Life Story: The Task of Reconciliation,' *Gerontologist* 3.2 (1999): 1373. See also Jerome Bruner, 'The Narrative Construction of Reality,' *Critical Inquiry* 18 (1991): 1–21; Norman Denzin, *Interpretive Biography* (Newbury Park, CA: Sage, 1989); Cheryl Mattingly, *Healing Dramas and Critical Plots: The Narrative Structure of Experience* (Cambridge, UK: Cambridge University Press, 1998).

> Could it be that there is a type of suffering that creates a new identity, the unknown identity of an unknown person who suffers? Could it be that cerebral suffering is precisely such suffering?[17]

Malabou's investigation of a combination of psychoanalytic and neurologic theories sheds light on problems of the brain such as dementia. At the heart of her definition of the problem lies trauma and a series of hypotheses that suggest 'patients with Alzheimer's disease or, more generally, patients with brain lesions, behave as if they are suffering from *war trauma*.'[18] Like traumatized soldiers, those suffering from dementia share disruptions in identity characterized by indifference and 'affective coolness.'[19] Theories of trauma, she argues, need to find ways of bridging the psychoanalytic and neurological assumptions of trauma. Until this happens, we are left with Malabou's own story:

> As for myself and the members of my family, we had no idea how to behave. We sat in the room, frightened, uncomprehending. We hastened to talk to my grandmother about 'normal' things, as if they would still have meaning for her. I understood too late that tenderness would have been the only way to respond; that the incoherence of my grandmother's behaviour and her visible indifference were also reactions to the shock of hospitalization.[20]

Whether the issue is the patient's absence or the family's incomprehension and fear of making the wrong decisions, dementia traumatizes. In the next section of this chapter I turn to storytelling as one way to confront the trauma to family and friends of those suffering from dementia.

5 Storytelling as a Way of Coping

I will never forget the morning the dreaded call came from the care facility. Mom had burned up a towel in her microwave and they found her sitting in the smoke, the window next to her chair still closed, not sure what she should do. Moves are never easy, on the patient or the family. When is it right? Will the change only make the confusion worse? Do we tell her or just bring her back to

---

17 Catherine Malabou, *The New Wounded: From Neurosis to Brain Damage* (New York: Fordham University Press, 2012), xii.

18 Ibid., xviii.

19 Ibid., xviii.

20 Ibid., xiv.

a new place? What's the old saying, 'Old age isn't for sissies'? Neither is having a family member with dementia. That day I knew she was no longer safe in an independent living facility, as regulated as it was. That realization did not help us determine the appropriate next facility. A lockdown memory unit seemed too extreme, group homes seemed more personalized but were mostly disappointing upon visitation, and assisted living felt short-term, too little too late. Dementia does not follow a timeline that helps families make these kinds of decisions. If we found these decisions daunting, what was it like for someone who had no contacts in social services for older adults?

Every time I returned from a bad visit I called Ken and Jan and their stories of living with parents with dementia were retold, embellished, matched – one of theirs with one of my own. Generally the shared storytelling worked, calming me down, helping me let go of the need to control. But sometimes telling stories is not enough, like the first time Mom forgot a family member.

> *When She Forgot Her Grandson*
> The forgetfulness and confusion steadily increased. One day my nephew came for a visit so I brought Mom to my house for dinner. She recognized the house immediately, although she didn't know who lived there. Jeff said, 'Hi Grandma.' She said 'Hi' and sat at the table ready to eat. In the middle of the meal she turned to me and asked who the man was sitting across from her. 'Mom, that's your grandson Jeff, Kristin's brother.' She replied, 'But he has curly dark hair and no one in my family looks like that.' 'Mom,' I replied, embarrassed for Jeff, 'Dad had black hair and Aunt Helen had curly black hair. Just because the boys and I had your blonde hair when we were kids doesn't mean no one in our family has dark hair.' 'Aunt Helen is his mother?' 'No Mom, Aunt Helen was Dad's sister. John and Sylvia are Jeff and Kristin's parents.' 'So John was married to Aunt Helen?' She looked across the table and remarked, 'Well he can't be part of my family. No one in my family is fat.' I tried to cover for the hurtful comment, 'Mom, the boys and I all fight our weight. Jeff is a Collins through and through.' Once we took Mom home Jeff said that left only his Mom's dad as a real grandparent, because he still knew him. Grandpa Les also has dementia, though as yet less severe.

To compound the pain of being forgotten, like many dementia patients, Mom has lost her social inhibitions. I did not know what to say to Jeff. I knew he was hurt. But whenever I walked into her room she would point to the pictures of her grandchildren, call them by name, tell me how proud she was of them. Jeff was hurt, but I was also hurt to think he had just given up on Mom because she was having one of her bad days. Mom and Jeff were both experiencing challenges to their identity. I hope she does not remember that she had claimed Jeff was not part of her family. Not everyone with dementia gets to forget their memory lapses. Family members certainly do not. What is it to be a child when the parent who knows you better than you know yourself is more and more frequently absent? Do you avoid seeing them, preferring to think of them as gone rather than getting your hopes up, thinking she is back because for five minutes everything has been as it used to be in that mythic time before dementia? As I told Jeanne the story of Mom and Jeff, she shared a story about her father.

> *I Hate the Way This Makes Me Feel*
> As my father reached his mid-eighties, he developed dementia. My brothers and I first realized it when Dad, clearly confused, could not tell us where he had been a few hours earlier. Then the day came that one of his friends called from downtown Little Rock to say that Dad was on his way home. He had been lost downtown, finally recognized a business that belonged to one of his friends, and stopped to ask for directions on how to get home. Now Dad stopped driving. He would walk around the apartment complex talking with people, making new friends, but he had lost his freedom, and was losing control of what had been crucial to him. One day he saw my brother (the oldest child) going over the family financial records beginning to prepare the taxes – something my father, a small business owner, had always done. Dad went to Mom and asked who that Ron person was that was going over the books.

The problem with this story and the ones I had been told along the same lines is that we all seek, in Arthur Frank's terms, a restitution story. We want a story that tells us how to make everything better – the way it was before the dementia. It isn't easy to talk about being forgotten, but at least stories bring the issue into the open. When friends tell stories about what it was like when this happened to them, they prepare those who have not faced it and fear the moment to come. Although these shared stories will not alleviate the shock when it happens to you, they help us know we are not alone.

Arthur Frank writes that '[s]erious illness is a loss of the "destination and map" that had previously guided the ill person's life: ill people have to learn "to think differently."'[21] So too do friends and family of those living with dementia. Frank goes on to argue that stories help the seriously ill forge a new destination and map: 'They learn by hearing themselves tell their stories, absorbing others'

21 Arthur W. Frank, *The Wounded Storyteller: Body, Illness, and Ethics* (Chicago: The University of Chicago Press, 1995), 1.

reactions, and experiencing their stories being shared.'[22] So too do stories help friends and family learn to cope with the ambiguity and helplessness of having a loved one suffer with dementia. Context changes the way a story is told and heard, and frequently the full lesson of the story is not apparent until you have experienced multiple times the behaviours that confuse or shock you. I still struggle with Mom's lack of social inhibitions. Instead of commenting on her grandson's weight, a mentally challenged girl's odd behaviour, or how ugly someone is, she has lately become obsessed with large breasts, including those of her new caregivers, and proclaims loudly and repeatedly, 'Look how huge they are; they must be uncomfortable.' My friend's stories mollify my embarrassment and I have learned subtle ways of moving Mom off this pattern of vocalization by remarking on the flowers in the garden or how pretty her newly polished nails look. Frank explains that we need to live with stories to make them our own, to absorb the lessons they offer. 'Thinking with stories ultimately requires a highly personal sedimentation of experience: living with the stories and having them shape perceptions of various experiences over time.'[23] Living with the stories I tell and those my friends tell me offers a form of control, of agency.

It makes a difference what kind of story is told. The restitution stories just postpone coming to terms with the perpetual ambiguity of living with the effects of dementia on a loved one. Frank offers two alternative story forms about illness. The first is the chaos story, told almost staccato where first one thing happened and then … and then …[24] This story form predominates when I call my brothers to report Mom's latest crisis. The telling is emotional venting, but it accomplishes little other than making them experience my frustration. A better choice is the quest narrative, described here from the perspective of the patient:

> Restitution stories attempt to outdistance mortality by rendering illness transitory. Chaos stories are sucked into the undertow of illness and the disasters that attend it. Quest stories meet suffering head on; they accept illness and seek to *use* it. Illness is the occasion of a journey that becomes a quest. What is quested may never be wholly clear, but the quest is defined by the ill person's belief that something is to be gained through the experience.[25]

Telling the quest story is an acknowledgment that something is gained through the experience of working through the trauma of dementia in a loved one.

22 Ibid., 1.
23 Ibid., 24.
24 Ibid., 98–99.
25 Ibid., 115.

Since we have no choice, trying to discover ways to live with the ambiguity seems the healthier option.

6 Conclusion

> *The Last Time*
> A year or so after Dad forgot my brother, I went home for Spring Break. It was the last time I saw Dad. The family had gathered in the apartment, but Dad had gone outside. I found him sitting on a bench – tired, and a little angry. He said sometimes he just wanted to take the car keys, drive away, and never come back; he hated the way this "sickness" made him feel. Dad knew what was happening to his mind; he had watched it happen to his older brother.

Living with a family member with dementia may not reach the level of PTSD, but the ambiguity of not knowing from moment to moment whether the person you knew or this new version of your loved one will appear is certainly a form of trauma. Each time the old familiar Mom appears, hope returns, unreasonable as I know it to be, that the old relationship and old identities can resume, that maybe this time I won't have to leave and hurry home to call a friend and begin again to cope by telling stories, and therein try to learn from the haunting reminder that life is not mine to control, but to experience, to learn from. Sharing stories helps me discover new ways of loving, and new ways of laughing with someone both here and gone. One final story seems appropriate. I was driving Mom to a doctor's appointment an hour away from her home. The day was rainy and I was having trouble seeing clearly. Mom said if I was tired maybe I shouldn't drive. I looked at her and asked if she thought it would be better if I pulled over and let her drive. After a moment she laughed realizing I was only kidding, that her days of driving were long past. For a moment our old bantering relationship was back. We both enjoyed it.

I am indebted to my storytelling circle, to Ken and Jan Nolley, Rollie and Dolores Wisbrock, Patricia Varas and Jeanne Clark who understand the steep learning curve for successfully coping with dementia in a parent, for discovering with me that telling stories helps provide relief, though not closure, from ambiguous loss, for understanding that obsessive repetition can be a very hostile form, but one we need to find humorous or tender rather than frustrating, and for reminding us that experiencing ambiguous loss may well prepare us for coping with the disease if we too must share our parent's fate. So it is fitting that I end as I began: Stories help us remember, and 'Memory implies a certain act of redemption. What is remembered has been saved from nothingness. What is forgotten is abandoned.'[26]

In loving memory of Wilma C. Collins, 28 September 1923 – 31 January 2016

Bibliography

Berger, John. *About Looking*. New York: Vintage International, 1980.

Boss, Pauline. 'The Trauma and Complicated Grief of Ambiguous Loss.' *Pastoral Psychology* 59 (2010): 137–145.

Bruner, Jerome. 'The Narrative Construction of Reality.' *Critical Inquiry* 18 (1991): 1–21.

Burke, Kenneth. *Counter-Statement*. Berkeley, CA: University of California Press, 1968.

Caruth, Cathy. *Trauma: Explorations in Memory*. Baltimore: Johns Hopkins University Press, 1995.

Cohen, Lawrence. 'Introduction: Thinking about Dementia.' *Thinking about Dementia: Cultural Loss and the Anthropology of Senility*, edited by Annette Leibing and Lawrence Cohen, 1–22. New Brunswick, NJ: Rutgers University Press, 2006.

Denzin, Norman. *Interpretive Biography*. Newbury Park, CA: Sage, 1989.

Fisher, Walter R. *Human Communication as Narration: Toward a Philosophy of Reason, Value, and Action*. Columbia SC: University of South Carolina Press, 1987.

Frank, Arthur W. *The Wounded Storyteller: Body, Illness, and Ethics*. Chicago: The University of Chicago Press, 1995.

Genette, Gérard. *Narrative Discourse: An Essay in Method*. Translated by Jane E. Lewin. Ithaca, New York: Cornell University Press, 1972.

Gubrium, Jaber and James Holstein. 'Narrative Practice and the Coherence of Personal Stories'. *Sociological Quarterly* 39.1 (1998): 163–187.

Hauerwas, Stanley. *A Community of Character: Towards a Constructive Christian Social Ethic*. Notre Dame, IN: University of Notre Dame Press, 1981.

Malabou, Catherine. *The New Wounded: From Neurosis to Brain Damage*. New York: Fordham University Press, 2012.

Mattingly, Cheryl. *Healing Dramas and Clinical Plots: The Narrative Structure of Experience*. Cambridge: Cambridge University Press, 1998.

McLean, Athena Helen. 'Coherence without Facticity in Dementia: The Case of Mrs. Fine.' *Thinking about Dementia: Culture, Loss, and the Anthropology of Senility*, edited by Annette Leibing and Lawrence Cohen, 157–169. New Brunswick, NJ: Rutgers University Press, 2006.

26 Berger, *About Looking*, 58.

CHAPTER 3

Young Children's Drawings after Sexual Abuse: Disclosure and Recovery

Elspeth McInnes

Abstract

Child sexual abuse is a contested social field where victims can face a range of risks arising from disclosure, including fear of threats and punishment by the perpetrator, lack of language or understanding to identify what has happened to them and the reactions of others, such as non-offending parents, police, child protection workers and educators. Unlike other forms of child abuse, child sexual abuse is always a criminal act, normally denied by alleged perpetrators, often involving investigations by child protection authorities and police. Disclosing sexual abuse can leave victims disbelieved, blamed for making such claims and isolated from safety and recovery processes. Despite these barriers, young children who are experiencing abuse can indirectly disclose what is happening to them through their behaviour and through drawings depicting their experiences. The interpretations placed on children's behaviour and the meanings attributed to their drawings are vulnerable to the beliefs of relevant adults, such as teachers, and their reactions. Improving educators' and other relevant professionals' abilities to interpret children's behaviours and drawings after abuse is important to improving the safety and recovery of victims. Using a collection of drawings from child victims the chapter identifies some common elements of abuse disclosures and the relationships between the drawings and the victims' emotional states. It briefly reviews some of the key behavioural differences marking normal and concerning behaviour of young children at school.

Keywords

disclosing child sexual abuse – drawings – schools – sexualised behaviour – teachers

1 Introduction

Despite community perceptions that child sexual abuse is rare and perpetrated by strangers who are social rejects, child sexual abuse is common, widespread,

 | DOI:10.1163/9789004397576_005

and most frequently enacted by a family member or another person known to the victim.[1] A community sample of Australian women found that one in five reported child sexual abuse, with half of these victims reporting vaginal or anal intercourse. Ninety-eight per cent of abusers reported in the research were males and 41 per cent were relatives. Seventy-one per cent of victims were under age twelve at the time of the abuse. Only 10 per cent of victims ever made a report to police or other authorities.[2]

In another major Australian population study, the Australian Bureau of Statistics Personal Safety Survey found that 12 per cent of women and 4.5 per cent of men said they were sexually abused before the age of fifteen.[3] Another Australian population study found that one in three women (33.6 per cent) and 15.9 per cent of men reported non-penetrative child sexual assaults whilst approximately 12 per cent of women and 4 per cent of men reported unwanted penetrative experiences.[4] Richardson and Bromfield report that most child sexual abuse is perpetrated by people who are known to the child, with an estimated ten to thirty per cent of cases involving strangers.[5] They also note that ninety per cent of child sexual abusers are male.

Although the population data on the prevalence of child sexual abuse reveals that the vast majority of child sexual abuse events are not reported to police, South Australian Police report data from 2000–1 revealed 952 reports of child sexual abuse. In nearly two in five incidents (38.8 per cent), the alleged perpetrator was a family member, with a parent figure accounting for a high proportion of these.[6] Eighty per cent of victims were female. Thirty-one per cent of victims were under age ten. Nine per cent of victims were under age five. Bearing in mind that Fleming's research found only one in ten victims make a report, these police data are likely to radically understate the extent of the problem, especially for young children whose language

1 Jan Breckenridge, 'An Exotic Phenomenon? Incest and Child Rape,' *Crimes of Violence: Australian Responses to Rape and Child Sexual Assault*, eds. Jan Breckenridge and Moira Carmody (Sydney: Allen and Unwin, 1992), 38.

2 Jane Fleming, 'Prevalence of Childhood Sexual Abuse in a Community Sample of Australian Women,' *Medical Journal of Australia* 166 (1997): 65.

3 Australian Bureau of Statistics, *Personal Safety Survey Catalogue Number 4906.0* (Canberra: AGPS, 2006), 12.

4 Michael P. Dunne, et al., 'Is Child Sexual Abuse Declining? Evidence from a Population-Based Survey of Men and Women in Australia,' *Child Abuse and Neglect* 27.2 (2003): 141–152.

5 Nick Richardson and Leah Bromfield, 'Who Abuses Children?' *Child Abuse Prevention Resource Sheet* 7 (Melbourne: Australian Institute of Family Studies, 2005).

6 Joy Wundersitz, *Child Sexual Assault Tracking from Police Incident Report to Finalisation in Court* (Adelaide: Office of Crime Statistics and Research, 2003).

and development inhibits their ability to comprehend and disclose their experience.[7]

Experiences of child sexual abuse victimisation have both short and long-term adverse effects, which vary with the age on onset, the frequency of victimisation, and the severity of the abuse.[8] Non-penetrative sexual abuse involving the child victim is linked with less severe consequences, however all victims experience adverse impacts to some degree. One-off instances of abuse by a stranger are more likely to be reported and the victim is more likely to be supported by authorities and family members, than cases that involve family members or trusted family associates.

A review of research into the short-term effects of child sexual abuse found that apart from sexualised behaviour, most short-term effects which were identified by the researchers included promiscuity by both male and female victims, boys expressing homosexual behaviour and an increased risk of re-victimization for both genders.[9] The researchers also noted increased rates of depression and suicidal ideation or behaviour amongst victims of child sexual abuse, compared to the general population and also compared to children diagnosed with a psychiatric condition who had not experienced child sexual abuse. Penetrative abuse, abuse using force or violence, and a close relationship with the perpetrator appeared to be the most harmful to child victims over time.[10]

Continuing exposure to sexual abuse is more likely to result in serious developmental and psychological problems for children, affecting their futures in multiple ways. Researchers have found these problems to include:
- disrupted attachment patterns affecting interpersonal relationships;
- disrupted emotional regulation and self-management;
- rapid behavioural regressions and shifting emotional states;
- anxiety and avoidance of social interaction and new experiences;
- absence of self-motivation and depression;
- aggressive behaviour toward the self and others;
- disregard of danger resulting in high-risk behaviours;
- self-hatred, self-blame and feelings of helpless ineffectiveness.[11]

---

7 Fleming, Prevalence of Childhood Sexual Abuse.

8 Rhys Price-Robertson, Penelope Rush, Liz Wall and Daryl Higgins, 'Rarely an Isolated Incident: Acknowledging the Inter-Relatedness of Child Maltreatment, Victimisation and Trauma,' *Child Family Community Australia* Paper 15 (2013), 3.

9 Joseph Beitchman, Kenneth Zucker, Jane Hood, Granville da Costa and Donna Akman, 'A Review of the Short-Term Effects of Child Sexual Abuse,' *Child Abuse and Neglect* 15 (1991): 537–556.

10 Ibid., 537.

11 Price-Robertson, Rush, Wall and Higgins, 'Rarely an Isolated Incident,' 7.

These responses to victimisation affect children's social relationships at home and at school and in later life, impacting on education and career and family prospects, affecting physical and mental health. A key risk factor is that victimisation can also result in children engaging in problem sexualised behaviour with other children, replicating their own trauma and affecting other children.[12] Although the research literature indicates that adult males who are known to the victim are the most common offenders in cases of child sexual assault, male children aged less than sixteen years are the second most common offender category.[13] Children as young as six years old have been reported for behaviours including touching of other children's genitals, oral sex and asking other children to engage in sexual behaviour with them.[14] Access to safety for the victims, support, therapy and recovery depends on the timely identification of child sexual abuse. This is important to reducing opportunities for abuse to continue unchecked as well as limiting the risk of the abuse affecting other children.

This chapter addresses the need to further educate professionals working with children to recognise indicators in children's drawings that they may be experiencing abuse. Teachers spend the most time with children after family members, positioning them as key agents in the process of identifying and reporting child abuse and supporting children's recovery after disclosure.[15]

2 Children Disclosing Abuse

As Mason identifies, disclosing sexualised trauma carries social costs for victims.[16] Apart from not having the language to speak about what has happened, many other factors inhibit children's disclosures of sexual abuse. Children are dependent on the care of adults and instructed to do as they are told. Their

12 Petra Staiger, *Children who Engage in Problem Sexualised Behaviours: Context, Characteristics and Treatment* (Ringwood Victoria: Australian Childhood Foundation, 2005).

13 Ian Nisbet, Sacha Rombouts and Stephen Smallbone, *Literature Review: Impacts of Programs for Adolescents who Sexually Offend* (Ashfield NSW: NSW Department of Community Services, 2005), iii.

14 Caroline Whitehouse, Fraser Gough, Sue Morwood and Cris Chapman, 'Lollies and Whistles: Beginnings and Endings with a Group for Children with Problematic Sexualised Behaviours' (paper presented at *Child Sexual Abuse: Justice Response or Alternative Resolution Conference*, Adelaide: Australian Institute of Criminology, 1–2 May 2003).

15 Freda Briggs, *Child Protection: The Essential Guide for Teachers and Other Professionals whose Work involves Children* (Docklands: JoJo Publishing, 2012), 54.

16 Anka Mason, in this volume.

knowledge of the world is limited and filtered through adults. Perpetrators are skilled at silencing children. These strategies include children being told that,

- the behaviours are secret and special between them;
- the behaviours are normal and an expression of love;
- no one would believe them;
- they are responsible for the abuse – they 'wanted it';
- another sibling would be assaulted if they refused;
- they are rude and bad, they would get into trouble and have to leave their family if they told anyone;
- they or loved ones (sometimes including the offender) would be harmed if they told;[17]
- their mother told him to do it to them.[18]

Hunter notes that responses to children's disclosures should be met with calm, careful, supportive listening and reassurances that they did the right thing to tell someone and let the child know what will happen next.[19] If a child does manage to say what has happened to them they would ideally be met with supportive acceptance, but common reactions variously include shock, denial, rejection or blame, especially when the alleged perpetrator is a family member or trusted friend or a person of authority and high social standing in institutional settings. There are many examples of social disbelief when religious leaders or celebrities, such as Australia's Rolf Harris, Britain's Jimmy Saville, or the United States' Penn State football coach Jerry Sandusky, have been exposed as prolific child sex offenders. Parents experience the same shock when the disclosure involves their partner, or other family member, trusted friend, neighbour, or authority figures such as church leaders or sporting coaches. Research by Hershkowitz, Lanes, and Lamb into victims' disclosure of child sexual abuse by non-family members, found that three in five parents tended to 'blame the children or act angrily.'[20] If the alleged perpetrator is a family member, the child will be vulnerable to their revenge for disclosing 'the secret.' Ullman's research also identified that negative reactions, such as disbelief, were

---

17 Freda Briggs with Michael McVeity, *Teaching Children to Protect Themselves* (Sydney: Allen & Unwin, 2000).

18 Anne Morris, 'The Mother of the Victim as Potential Supporter and Protector: Considerations and Challenges' (paper presented at *Child Sexual Abuse: Justice Response or Alternative Resolution Conference*, Adelaide: Australian Institute of Criminology, 1–2 May 2003).

19 Cathryn Hunter, 'Responding to Children and Young People's Disclosures of Abuse,' *Practice Brief* (Melbourne: National Child Protection Clearinghouse, 2011).

20 Irit Hershkowtiz, Omer Lanes and Michael E. Lamb, 'Exploring the Disclosure of Child Sexual Abuse with Alleged Victims and Their Parents,' *Child Abuse and Neglect* 31.2 (2007): 111.

observed more often for those victimized by relatives compared with stranger or acquaintance victims, especially if they disclosed during childhood.[21] Child sexual abuse by a family member provides a context where abuse of a child is likely to be repetitive and continue over months and years, unlike stranger or acquaintance abuse, which is typically opportunistic.[22] Family member child sex offenders affect relationships within the family and, in cases where the offender is the primary income earner, the child's disclosures could result in the family becoming impoverished if the offender is imprisoned. The level of maternal support available to children who have been sexually abused has been found to have a significant positive mediating effect on later psychopathology.[23]

Hunter defines disclosure as a process rather than an event.[24] She notes that some children may initially deny abuse then later disclose, or disclose and then retract the disclosure as a result of the consequent stress. McElvaney, Greene and Hogan argue that sexually abused children struggle with containing the secret of their abuse, wanting at once to reveal what has happened but being fearful of the consequences threatened by their abuser. They describe a process first of the victim coming to terms with how they feel about what has happened and the decision to tell, followed by an 'active-withholding dynamic' about when and how to tell, who to tell and how to manage the consequences of disclosure.[25] Such caution is entirely reasonable when it is remembered that, in the absence of corroborating forensic evidence, such as an adult witness or DNA evidence, the alleged perpetrator will likely not be prosecuted, but the child's disclosures will be made known to the perpetrator by investigators. When disclosures are reported to police, the police interview process itself can re-traumatize the child and may not lead to charges if police consider the child a poor witness.[26] Research into police beliefs about how children

---

21 Sarah Ullman, 'Relationship to Perpetrator, Disclosure, Social Reactions and PTSD Symptoms in Child Sexual Abuse Survivors,' *Journal of Child Sexual Abuse* 16 (2007): 19.

22 Stephen Smallbone and Richard Wortley, 'Child Sexual Abuse: Offender Characteristics and Modus Operandi,' *Trends and Issues in Crime and Criminal Justice* (Canberra: Australian Institute of Criminology, 2001), 193.

23 Kathleen Kendall-Tackett, Linda Meyer Williams and David Finkelhor, 'Impact of Sexual Abuse on Children: A Review and Synthesis of Recent Empirical Studies,' *Psychological Bulletin* 113 (1993): 164–180.

24 Hunter, *Responding to Children*, 4–6.

25 Rosaleen McElvaney, Sheila Greene and Diane Hogan, 'Containing the Secret of Child Sexual Abuse,' *Journal of Interpersonal Violence* 27.6 (2012): 1170.

26 Christine Eastwood, 'The Experiences of Child Complainants of Sexual Abuse in the Criminal Justice System,' *Trends & Issues in Crime and Criminal Justice* (Canberra: Australian Institute of Criminology, 2003), 250.

report abuse identified that the characteristics on which police interviewers made judgements of credibility were not reliable, resulting in decisions no better than chance as to whether they assessed children as credible witnesses to their abuse or not.[27] Faced with the repercussions of disclosure from family, child protection, and criminal justice systems, victims can feel trapped with their secret. A review of research with sexually abused children identified that involvement in court proceedings often had an adverse impact on their recovery from the abuse.[28] Children were worst affected when they had to testify in court on multiple occasions, particularly when their testimony was harshly challenged and they were afraid of the offender.

There can also be adverse consequences for victims arising from delayed disclosure. Sinclair and Gold's research with adults who were sexually abused as children and who delayed disclosure, found that victims enduring more severe abuse were more likely to delay fully disclosing the abuse and that such delay was associated with more trauma-related symptoms.[29]

Despite the obstacles to disclosure, children can indirectly reveal experiences of sexual abuse through comments, questions, or drawings. Drawing is a way for children to express their perceptions and emotions, often with commentary about what is happening in the picture.[30] It is a common activity in preschool and junior primary classrooms to invite children to draw events such as family holidays, their favourite activities, or even more complex concepts such as school rules. Given that Australia has compulsory education from age five and access to pre-school from age four, young children who have been sexually abused are among the population of children creating drawings in education settings. It is important that educators are able to recognise signifiers, which deserve further scrutiny.

3 Children's Drawings after Sexual Abuse

Research by Jacobs-Kayam, Lev-Wiesel and Zohar found that drawings of themselves by adolescents who had previously been sexually abused, revealed

27 Carolyn Hughes-Scholes, Martine B. Powell and Stefanie J. Sharman. 'An Examination of Police Officers' Beliefs about how Children Report Abuse,' *Psychiatry, Psychology and Law* 21.1 (2013): 127–138. DOI:10.1080/13218719.2013.793153.

28 Kendall-Tackett, Williams and Finkelhor, 'Impact of Sexual Abuse on Children,' 170.

29 Barbara Sinclair and Steven Gold, 'The Psychological Impact of Withholding Disclosure of Child Sexual Abuse,' *Violence and Victims* 12 (1997): 137–45.

30 Freda Briggs and Karen Lehmann, 'The Significance of Children's Drawings in Cases of Child Sexual Abuse,' *Early Childhood Development and Care* 47 (1989): 133.

indicators of child sexual abuse and self-harming behaviour in adolescents. Indicators included an incomplete or emphasised face line, often missing features, blank eyes, missing hands and arms, and with emphasised genitals.[31] Shiakou's research found that family drawings by maltreated children aged five to eleven showed evidence of insecure attachment, with the child depicted alone or apart from their family in contrast to the drawings by non-maltreated children, who always drew themselves with their family.[32]

Patterson and Hayne researched whether drawing about an event increased the amount of information children provide during an interview.[33] They tested 90 five- to twelve-year-old children who were asked to draw emotional events they experienced. The researchers found that drawing had no negative effect on the accuracy of children's accounts, and it increased the information children provided about events, as well as providing cues to interviewers about questions to ask. Katz and Hamama similarly found that drawings enabled sexually abused children to provide more details and speak more coherently about what had happened to them.[34] Macleod, Gross and Hayne found that five- to twelve-year-old children were able to give more details about their thoughts and emotions using interactive draw and tell techniques. These techniques involved the researchers directing children to draw and describe specific experiences, followed by prompting questions such as 'what happened?' or 'what is it?' or 'where did you see that?'[35] Drawing and telling provides a strategy to overcome children's language limitations, both developmentally, and in terms of the vocabulary to accurately name and describe what has happened to them. Young children often have limited knowledge of the correct names of body parts or the names of sexual acts, which can make it difficult for adults to understand what has happened to the victim. In any subsequent criminal proceedings the quality of evidence relies on the ability of victims to recall

31 Angi Jacobs-Kayam, Rachel Lev-Wiesel and Gail Zohar, 'Self-Mutilation as Expressed in Self-Figure Drawings in Adolescent Sexual Abuse Survivors,' *The Arts in Psychotherapy* 40 (2013): 120.

32 Monica Shiakou, 'Representations of Attachment Patterns in the Family Drawings of Maltreated and non-Maltreated Children,' *Child Abuse Review* 21 (2012): 203.

33 Tess Patterson and Harlene Hayne, 'Does Drawing Facilitate Older Children's Reports of Emotionally Laden Events?' *Applied Cognitive Psychology* 25 (2011): 119.

34 Carmit Katz and Liat Hamama, 'Draw Me Everything that Happened to You: Exploring Young Children's Drawings of Sexual Abuse,' *Children and Youth Services Review* 35 (2013): 877.

35 Emily Macleod, Julien Gross and Harlene Hayne, 'The Clinical and Forensic Value of Information that Children Report while Drawing,' *Applied Cognitive Psychology* 27 (2013): 565.

and recount their experiences. Drawings can also provide a way for victims of child sexual abuse to identify and process what has happened to them as part of a therapeutic process. Perpetrators' silencing strategies include making the victim feel responsible for what happened to them.[36] Making a drawing of the abuse enables the victim to depict the event, and the responsibility, as external to themselves.

Allen and Tussey reviewed research to determine whether specific graphic indicators or scoring systems could reliably distinguish between abused and non-abused children, and found that no indicator or system reliably indicated abuse.[37] Allen and Tussey's research highlights the need to explore children's drawings in conversation with the artists, rather than leaping to a conclusion based on any single indicator of concern. Drawings will inevitably vary in ways that preclude any singular analysis. The graphic indicators examined by Allen and Tussey included depiction of genitalia and omission of body parts. These features have been identified in the literature as indicators of potential sexual abuse, deserving further scrutiny and questioning.[38]

Junior Primary School Teachers are commonly exposed to children's drawings in the course of day-to-day classroom activities. The universal provision of primary school education means that teachers are the professional group most likely to have regular contact with children after their parents and other family members. They are therefore a key professional group needing to develop their ability to identify pictures that indicate a need for further inquiry.[39] Children's drawings develop alongside other academic skills, such as reading and writing, showing greater details and complexities as they develop. The following two drawings provide examples of art by six-year-old children when asked to draw a school rule.[40]

The two pictures in Figures 3.1 and 3.2 clearly depict children breaking the selected rule detailed in each picture. In each of these drawings the child artist has used a wide range of colours. Note the use of red for danger as the colour of the sand being directed at the child's head in Figure 3.1. It is also worth noting that both drawings depict a smiling offender and a sad victim, showing

36 Smallbone and Wortley, 'Child Sexual Abuse,' 4.

37 Brian Allen and Chriscelyn Tussey, 'Can Projective Drawings Detect if a Child Experienced Sexual or Physical Abuse? A Systemic Review of the Controlled Research,' *Trauma, Violence Abuse* 13.2 (2012): 97.

38 Briggs, *Child Protection: The Essential Guide*, 220.

39 Ibid., 54.

40 All drawings and information about them have been extracted from the teaching collection used by the author to inform pre-service early childhood educators. They have been collected from parents and professionals responding to young children.

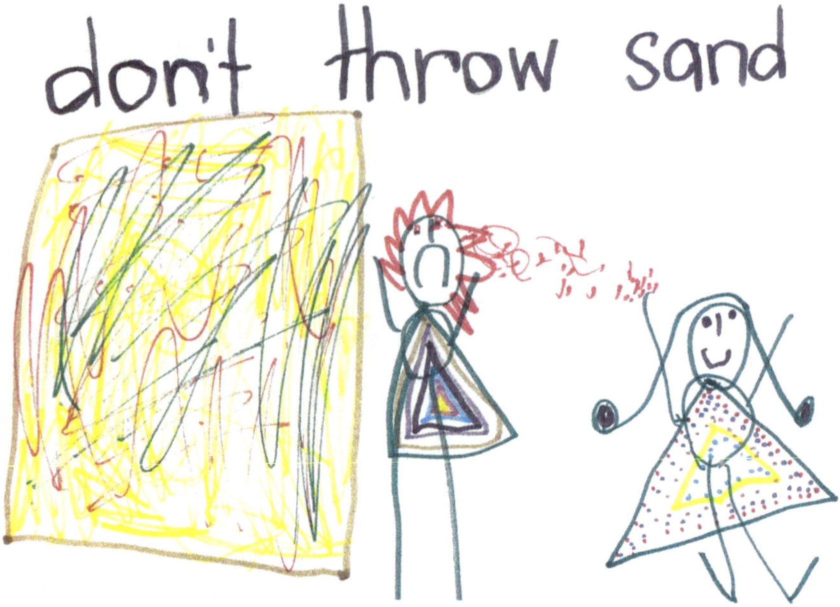

FIGURE 3.1 Drawing of school rules: *Don't Throw Sand*

children's awareness of the emotional impacts of the behaviour depicted. The sad face of the victim reflects an awareness of the adverse impact on them. Conversely the smiling face of the child who is breaking the rule appears to reflect a view that the action of throwing sand or playing with sticks is an enjoyable one for the rule-breaker. Note also that all human figures are fully represented, fully clothed, with no visible genitals, standing on the ground with arms and legs and all facial features. These details can be contrasted with the images in the following drawings by children of a similar age, where children variously represent themselves and others with visible genitals, with body parts and facial features exaggerated or missing.

The drawing skills of children who have been abused often regress into less developed depictions than they had previously been drawing. Figure 3.3 was presented to a teacher by the eight-year-old artist who stated, 'This is a man with his trousers down and that's his dick up to his chin.'

The picture shows a rudimentary body shape and a prominent oval shaped mouth with exaggerated jagged teeth. Unlike the human figures in Figures 3.1 and 3.2, the man shown in Figure 3.3 has no ears or hair or nose. The feet and hands do not resemble actual fingers or toes. Like the rule-breakers in the previous drawings, the man appears to be smiling. The depictions of large, open

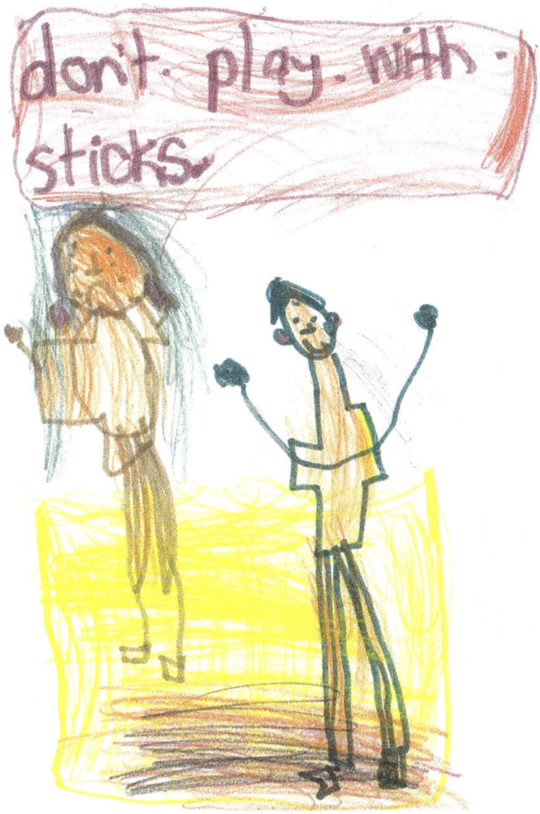

FIGURE 3.2 Drawing of school rules: *Don't Play With Sticks*

mouths with teeth are often featured in drawings by children who have been exposed to oral sex. The oversize genitals in Figure 3.3 can be understood as a child's eye view of an adult erect penis. Young children's small size relative to adults means that adults are often depicted as disproportionately large. When asked what she said to the artist in response to his description of his drawing, the teacher replied 'Nothing. I was just too embarrassed.'

There were a number of indicators of concern that something was affecting the child's well-being, warranting further attention from school staff. The boy had previously been transferred to the school's special education unit because his engagement in school work had been well behind his class mates in the mainstream classroom. The Principal later revealed the child had previously been brought to her by another teacher after he had been found sexually

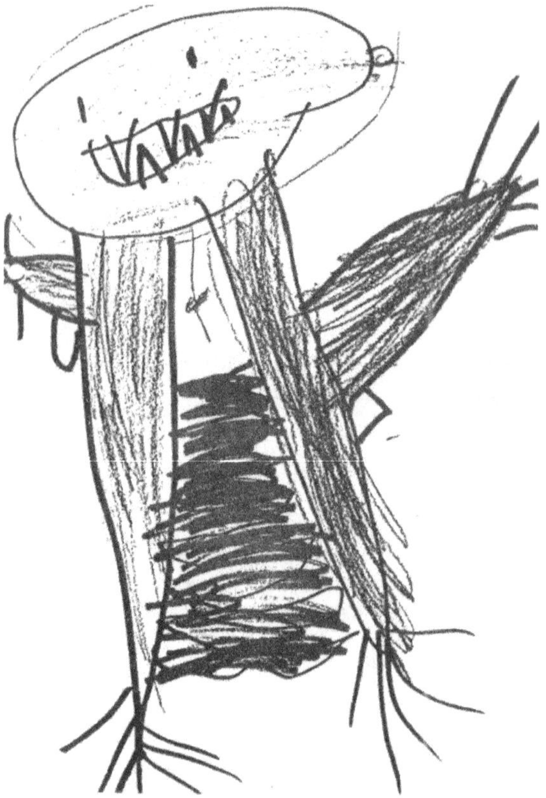

FIGURE 3.3 Drawing after sexual abuse: *Tooth-Faced Man*

abusing other children in the toilets. The Principal had responded by keeping him indoors at recess for a week. No report to child protection was ever made, despite state legislation mandating that educators must report reasonable suspicions of child abuse to child protection authorities. The boy continued to be abused and to abuse others because of the teacher's embarrassment and the Principal's failure to recognise the significance of the boy's coercive sexual conduct in relation to other younger children.

If the teacher had responded to the artist's statement with the questions such as, 'Who is this in your picture?' or 'Where did you see that?' the child may have been able to provide information sufficient to make a mandatory report. In any case, the child's coercive sexual abuse of other younger children should have been reported to child protection authorities. The seriousness of the child's behaviour and its indications that the child may have been subjected

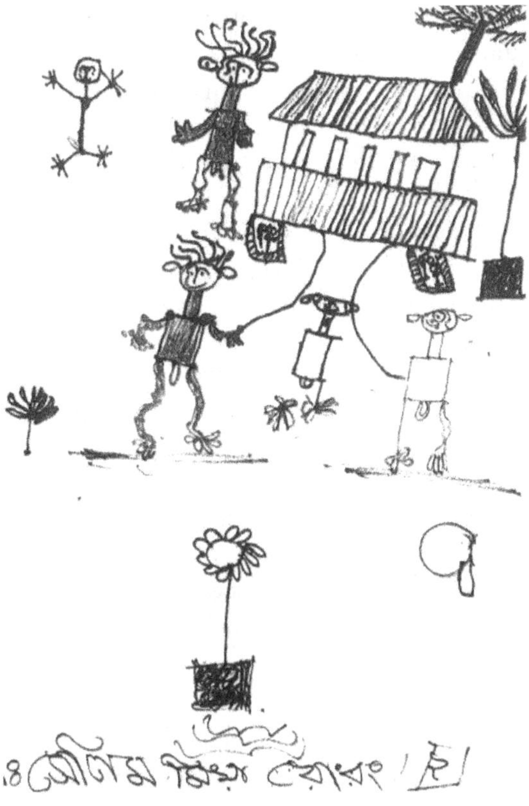

FIGURE 3.4 Drawing after sexual abuse: *Bangladesh School*

to similar behaviour was not recognised by the school's leadership. Too often, such indicators are trivialised or dismissed as normal sexual curiosity and simply discouraged.[41] Such responses breach mandatory reporting laws and fail to address the needs of the child perpetrator and his victims, increasing the risk that the child will continue his sexually abusive conduct towards other children.

Graffiti in schools is common, with many school toilet walls adorned with drawings of male genitals. Typically these drawings are disembodied, yet their frequency can disarm educators from recognising a problem. In Figure 3.4, a children's charity built a school in Bangladesh and the children sent pictures

41 Staiger, *Children who Engage in Problem Sexualised Behaviours*, 22.

to thank the Board. Most of the drawings showed an obsession with genitals. The Board dismissed the ubiquitous depiction of genitals as 'boys will be boys,' but learned later that the children had been rescued from child brothels. The attention given to genitals reflected the child's experiences of brothel customers' focus. Again, the Board did not recognise the risk that child victims would replicate the behaviour with other children.

Figure 3.5 also features an emphasis on genitals. The child artist was later found to have been sexually abused by a family friend. As with previous pictures featuring genitals, it was not noticed by the teacher as raising any concerns. As with previous illustrations, the mouth is very prominent but the face lacks important details.

The following drawing in Figure 3.6 was done by a seven-year-old girl during therapy, depicting the details of her abuse. The liberal use of colour in the picture contrasts with the heavy dark tones of many children's drawings depicting abuse. The use of bright colours could be a consequence of the child attending therapy at the time the picture was drawn. The therapeutic environment may have assisted her to process some of the feelings about her sexual abuse experiences.

The picture is quite detailed and the figures of the offender and victim are complete with arms, hands, fingers, legs and feet. The explicit depiction of fellatio is the dominant detail. As in other drawings by children who have been sexually abused, the penis size is drawn as enormous and greatly disproportionate. The mouth size of the victim is also featured with exaggerated teeth, while the offender is shown as smiling and happy. As was noted in relation to Figure 3.3, exaggerated mouths and teeth are common in depictions of oral sex. This drawing was produced for a psychologist after a series of events in which the child had disclosed, been interviewed and medically assessed, and believed by child protection services and a paediatrician, and was living safely with her mother. The perpetrator father applied for custody in the Family Court that held that the mother had coached the child to make false allegations and, therefore, the child should live with the father. The mother fled overseas to protect her children. They were located and the children placed in an institution for a year before being returned to foster care placements in Australia under the Hague Convention on Child Abduction. After some years without their mother, they were allowed to return to her care but were both suffering from mental illnesses.

The artwork in Figure 3.7 (below) is that of a seven-year-old girl who was being abused by her mother and older brother. At school she presented as sad and withdrawn. Again the perpetrators are depicted as smiling, enjoying what they are doing. The mother is shown as a large animal, much larger than the victim, whilst the brother has a phallic shape. The victim's self-portrait shows her as

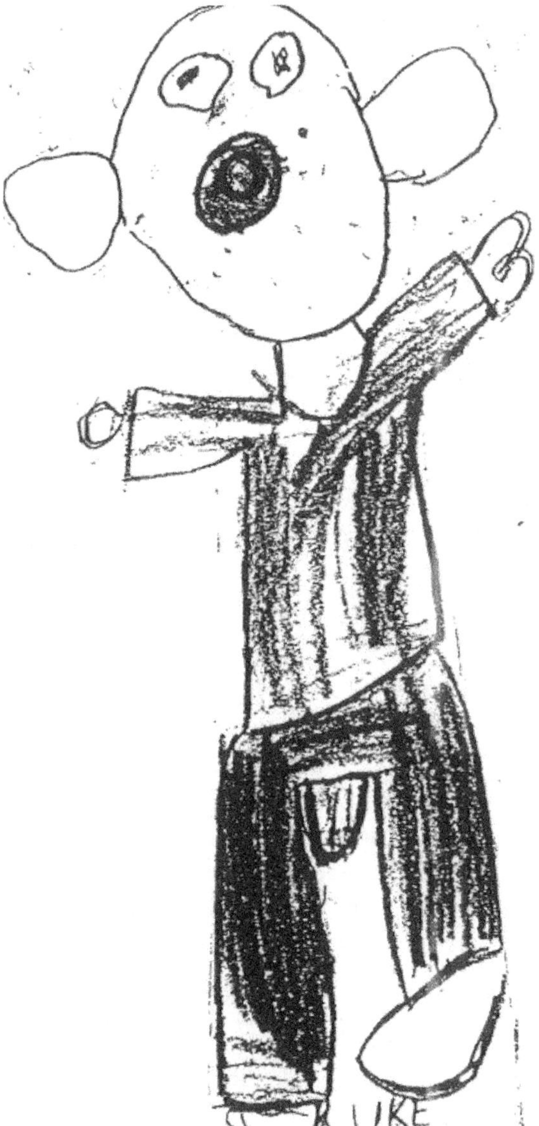

FIGURE 3.5 Drawing after sexual abuse: *Luke's Picture*

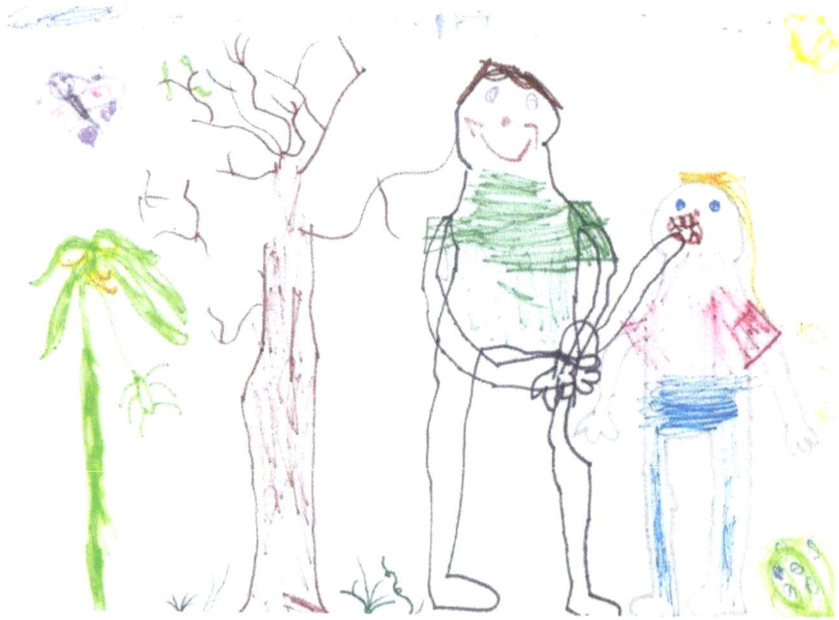

FIGURE 3.6 Drawing after sexual abuse: *Father-Daughter*

armless and faceless, floating in limbo, in contrast to the other figures, which are depicted with feet on the ground. The absence of a face and mouth points to her absence of voice and identity. The absence of arms depicts her helplessness. She floats above the ground, unconnected, much the same as a dissociation experience, reported by many child sex abuse victims as a coping strategy during the abuse experience. Research by Amir and Lev-Weisel has also identified the depiction of dissociation in the drawings of child sexual abuse victims.[42] The child's writing is incoherent, but the teacher has scripted her statement 'My family is good' about the picture. Again the teacher accepted the picture at face value and did not ask her about what was happening in the picture.

Figure 3.8 is the artwork of a four-year-old girl who was sexually abused by a man when she went to the toilet at a neighbour's barbecue. She told her mother that the bad man hurt her. She was believed. There was no secret, no breach

42 Galit Amir and Rachel Lev-Wiesel, 'Dissociation as Depicted in the Traumatic Event Drawings of Child Sexual Abuse Survivors: A Preliminary Study,' *The Arts in Psychotherapy* 34 (2007): 114.

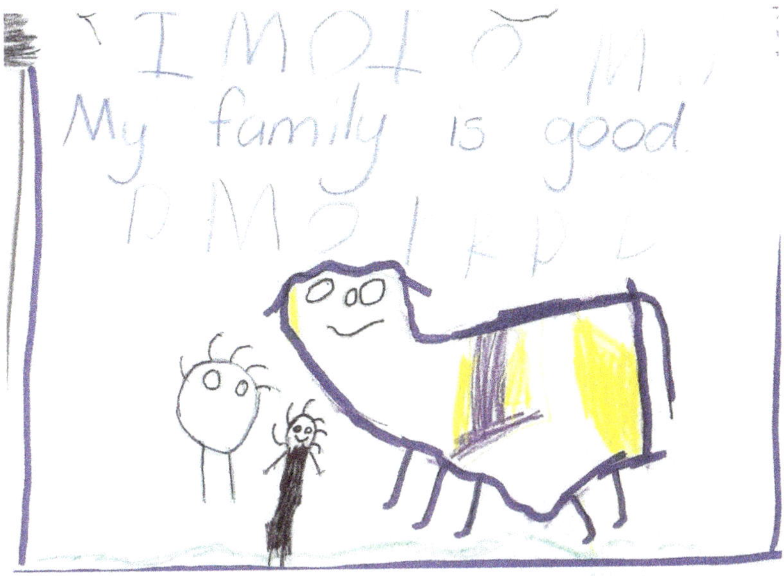

FIGURE 3.7 Drawing after sexual abuse: *My Family is Good*

of trust, no secret, no threats BUT, the following day she started drawing herself without arms.

Figure 3.9 is the same child's picture of the man who abused her. His figure features arms and legs. The arms are very large with long sharp fingers. The mouth and eyes are also large. Her perspective as a small child emphasises the size of the arms that grabbed her and his face up close to her face. Each figure features a hole in the middle of the body.

Figure 3.10 is the child's self-portrait after therapy. In order to gain a sense of mastery over her attacker, the therapist asked the child to draw a picture of the bad man then chop it up with scissors. The symbolic destruction of the perpetrator depicted in the child's artwork enabled the victim to reconstruct her relationship to the man who attacked her. During the attack, the relative size of the perpetrator, the surprise of finding him hiding in the toilet, his purposeful knowledge and intent towards the victim, and the absence of any supportive adult had removed any sense of control over what was happening to her. By cutting the image of her attacker into pieces, the child was able to exercise her control over the perpetrator and literally 'destroy' his hold over her. The sense of helplessness and lack of control during the attack had translated into anxiety after the attack that her experiences of abuse could be repeated at any time. By symbolically taking back her control over her attacker, the victim was

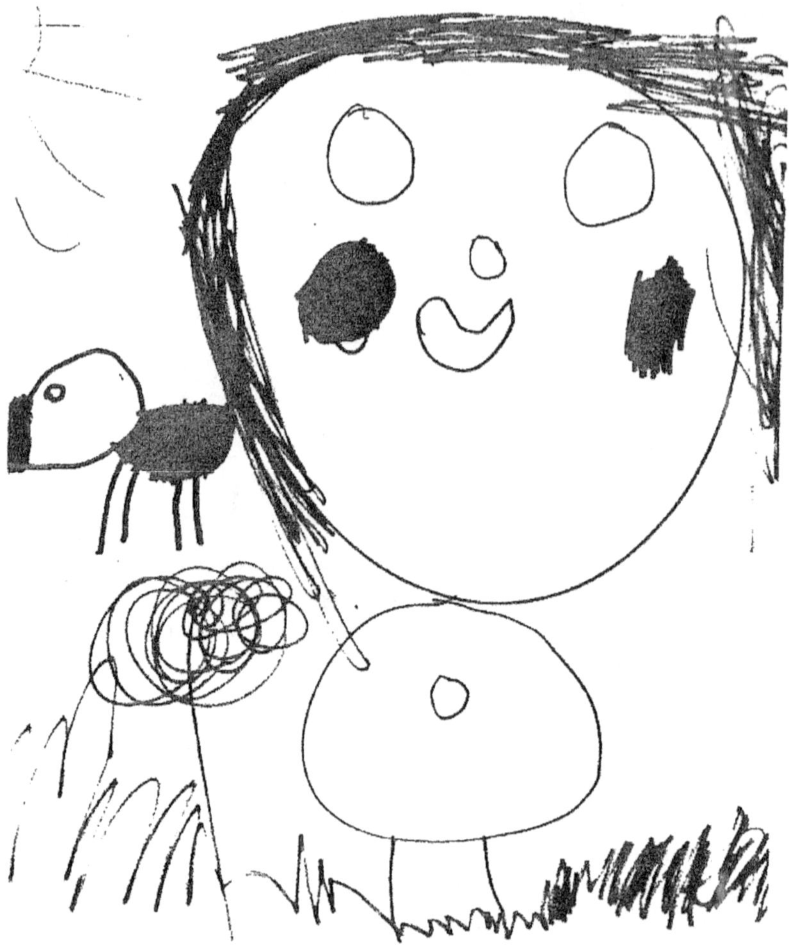

FIGURE 3.8 Drawing after sexual abuse: *Empty Eye Victim*

empowered to believe herself to again be safe and supported. Her subsequent drawing of herself showed a noticeable change in her self-image. She has arms and legs, she is smiling and her eyes are coloured in, no longer empty.

4 Discussion

Disclosure of child sexual abuse is a difficult process for victims, with many children delaying revealing the abuse for a long time. Lack of knowledge of

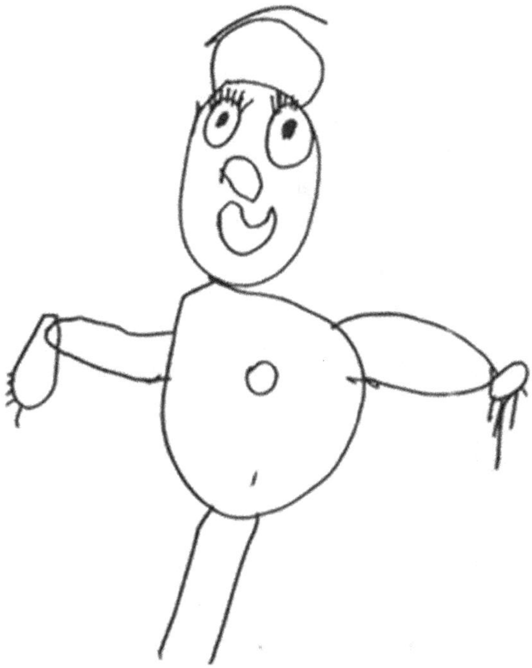

FIGURE 3.9 Drawing after sexual abuse: *Perpetrator*

what has happened to them, lack of language to speak about it, fear of disclosing and fear of the consequences of disclosure, keep victims silent and vulnerable to continuing abuse and isolated from help and protection. Preying on victims' fears of what would happen to them and their loved ones if they disclosed is a favoured strategy used by offenders to avoid detection and to continue to have access to their victims. The drawings of children who have been sexually abused can however provide indicators that responsible adults in the child's life should ask open-ended questions about their drawings. Spontaneous or prompted statements by the artists about their pictures should be documented and dated. Explicit disclosures need to be reported to relevant child protection and police authorities. Such actions will only be taken however, if relevant professionals are alert to the issue and know how to respond.

Systemic reforms are needed to better inform professionals about the indicators, dynamics, impacts and consequences of child sexual abuse. The traumatising impacts on children's wellbeing and their development need to be better understood by educators, social workers, police, lawyers and

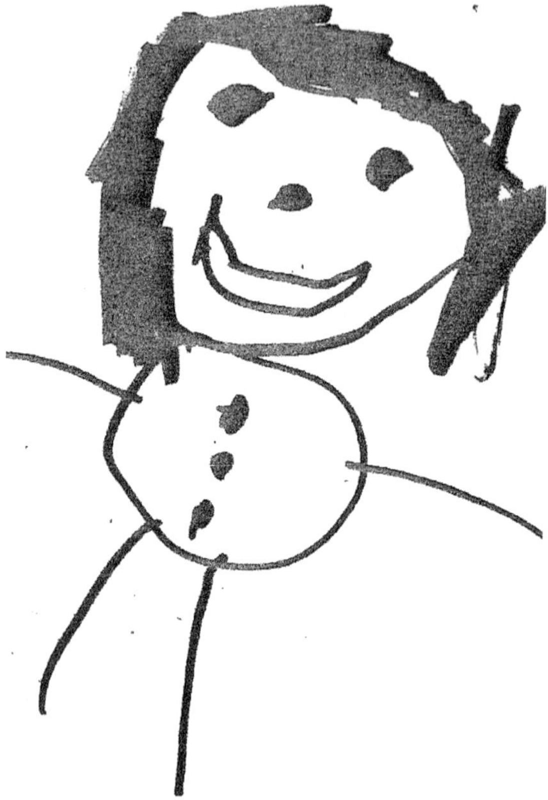

FIGURE 3.10 Drawing after sexual abuse: *Recovery Smile*

other professionals who have a role in detecting and responding to child sexual abuse. The availability of professional expertise in child development and trauma is a constant problem in systems that are primarily designed around adult needs and concepts.

Building capacity amongst relevant professionals to identify and respond to child sexual abuse is a constant challenge, particularly because child sexual abuse is such an abhorrent crime. In a classroom context, drawings can provide important clues for educators and carers to look more closely and ask more questions of children whose drawings feature indicators of sexual abuse. There are different depictions of the perpetrators and the victims that may be represented separately or in the same picture. As the drawings in this chapter illustrate, pictures of perpetrators often include genitals, particularly large penises or phallic shapes, large mouths with teeth, large arms and hands and fingers. They may be shown with smiling faces and in dark colours. The victim is often pictured as small, incomplete, lacking facial features, missing arms or legs, floating in limbo, whereas the child had previously been able to draw these features.

Because many victims have been frightened, tricked or induced to keep the secret of their abuse, they may avoid speaking directly about what has happened to them, but feel able to talk about the picture. Asking open questions such as 'tell me what is in this picture?' 'Who is this?' 'Where did you learn about that?' can support the child to give enough details for the teacher to make a report. Teachers and other human services professionals working with children can benefit from learning strategies to elicit children's drawings and the knowledge to discern when they should inquire further.

Drawings have also proven to be valuable in forensic and therapeutic settings, with children who have already been identified as abused, as they enable children to give more coherent detail of what has happened, providing useful prompts for interviewers. Paying attention to the content and form of children's drawings can result in the abuse being identified and stopped and the victim having access to support and recovery.

Bibliography

Allen, Brian, and Chriscelyn Tussey. 'Can Projective Drawings Detect if a Child Experienced Sexual or Physical Abuse? A Systemic Review of the Controlled Research.' *Trauma, Violence Abuse* 13.2 (2009): 97–111.

Amir, Galit, and Rachel Lev-Wiesel. 'Dissociation as Depicted in the Traumatic Event Drawings of Child Sexual Abuse Survivors: A Preliminary Study.' *The Arts in Psychotherapy* 34 (2007): 114–123.

Australian Bureau of Statistics. *Personal Safety Survey, Catalogue Number 4906.0*. Canberra: AGPS, 2006.

Beitchman, Joseph, Kenneth Zucker, Jane Hood, Granville da Costa and Donna Akman. 'A Review of the Short-Term Effects of Child Sexual Abuse.' *Child Abuse and Neglect* 15 (1991): 537–556.

Breckenridge, Jan. 'An Exotic Phenomenon? Incest and Child Rape.' *Crimes of Violence: Australian Responses to Rape and Child Sexual Assault*, edited by Jan Breckenridge and Moira Carmody, 37–61. Sydney: Allen and Unwin, 1992.

Briggs, Freda. *Child Protection: The Essential Guide for Teachers and Other Professionals whose Work involves Children*. JoJo Publishing: Docklands, 2012.

Briggs, Freda, with Michael McVeity. *Teaching Children to Protect Themselves*. Sydney: Allen & Unwin, 2000.

Briggs, Freda and Karen Lehmann. 'The Significance of Children's Drawings in Cases of Child Sexual Abuse.' *Early Childhood Development and Care* 47 (1989): 131–147.

Dunne, Michael P., David M. Purdie, Michelle D. Cook, Frances M. Boyle and Jake M. Najman. 'Is Child Sexual Abuse Declining? Evidence from a Population-Based Survey of Men and Women in Australia.' *Child Abuse and Neglect* 27.2 (2003): 141–152.

Eastwood, Christine. 'The Experiences of Child Complainants of Sexual Abuse in the Criminal Justice System.' *Trends & Issues in Crime and Criminal Justice* 250 Canberra: Australian Institute of Criminology, 2003.

Fleming, Jane. 'Prevalence of Childhood Sexual Abuse in a Community Sample of Australian Women.' *Medical Journal of Australia* 166 (1997): 65–68.

Hershkowtiz, Irit, Omer Lanes and Michael E. Lamb. 'Exploring the Disclosure of Child Sexual Abuse with Alleged Victims and their Parents.' *Child Abuse and Neglect* 31.2 (2007): 111–123.

Hughes-Scholes, Carolyn, Martine B. Powell and Stefanie J. Sharman. 'An Examination of Police Officers' Beliefs about how Children Report Abuse.' *Psychiatry, Psychology and Law* 21.1 (2013): 127–138. DOI:10.1080/13218719.2013.793153.

Hunter, Kathryn. 'Responding to Children and Young People's Disclosures of Abuse.' *Practice Brief.* Melbourne: National Child Protection Clearinghouse, 2011.

Jacobs-Kayam, Angi, Rachel Lev-Wiesel and Gail Zohar. 'Self-Mutilation as Expressed in Self-Figure Drawings in Adolescent Sexual Abuse Survivors.' *The Arts in Psychotherapy* 40 (2013): 120–129.

Katz, Carmit and Liat Hamama. 'Draw Me Everything that Happened to You: Exploring Young Children's Drawings of Sexual Abuse.' *Children and Youth Services Review* 35 (2013): 877–882.

Kendall-Tackett, Kathleen, Linda Meyer Williams and David Finkelhor. 'Impact of Sexual Abuse on Children: A Review and Synthesis of Recent Empirical Studies.' *Psychological Bulletin* 113 (1993):164–180.

Macleod, Emily, Julien Gross and Harlene Hayne. 'The Clinical and Forensic Value of Information that Children Report While Drawing.' *Applied Cognitive Psychology* 27 (2013): 564–573.

McElvaney, Rosaleen, Sheila Greene and Diane Hogan. 'Containing the Secret of Child Sexual Abuse.' *Journal of Interpersonal Violence* 27.6 (2012): 1155–1175.

Morris, Anne. 'The Mother of the Victim as Potential Supporter and Protector: Considerations and Challenges.' Paper presented at *Child Sexual Abuse: Justice Response or Alternative Resolution Conference.* Adelaide: Australian Institute of Criminology, 1–2 May 2003.

Nisbet, Ian, Sacha Rombouts and Stephen Smallbone. *Literature Review: Impacts of Programs for Adolescents who Sexually Offend.* Ashfield NSW: NSW Department of Community Services, 2005.

Patterson, Tess and Harlene Hayne. 'Does Drawing Facilitate Older Children's Reports of Emotionally Laden Events?' *Applied Cognitive Psychology* 25 (2011): 119–126.

Price-Robertson, Rhys, Penelope Rush, Liz Wall and Daryl Higgins. 'Rarely an Isolated Incident: Acknowledging the Inter-Relatedness of Child Maltreatment, Victimisation and Trauma.' *Child Family Community Australia* Paper 15 (2013).

Richardson, Nick and Leah Bromfield. 'Who Abuses Children?' *Child Abuse Prevention Resource Sheet* 7. Melbourne: Australian Institute of Family Studies, 2005.

Sinclair, Barbara and Steven Gold. 'The Psychological Impact of Withholding Disclosure of Child Sexual Abuse.' *Violence and Victims* 12 (1997): 137–145.

Shiakou, Monica. 'Representations of Attachment Patterns in the Family Drawings of Maltreated and Non-Maltreated Children.' *Child Abuse Review* 21 (2012): 203–218.

Smallbone, Stephen and Richard Wortley. 'Child Sexual Abuse: Offender Characteristics and Modus Operandi.' *Trends and Issues in Crime and Criminal Justice* Paper 193. Canberra: Australian Institute of Criminology, 2001.

Staiger, Petra. *Children who Engage in Problem Sexualised Behaviours: Context, Characteristics and Treatment.* Ringwood, Victoria: Australian Childhood Foundation, 2005.

Ullman, Sarah. 'Relationship to perpetrator, Disclosure, Social Reactions, and PTSD Symptoms in Child Sexual Abuse Survivors.' *Journal of Child Sexual Abuse* 16 (2007): 19–36.

CHAPTER 4

Resiliency, a Mediator between War Experience and Aggressive Behaviour

Rana Tayara

Abstract

During the Lebanese and Israeli war of July 2006, Lebanese adolescents had been exposed to numerous traumatic events such as shelling, displacement, witnessing violence, injuries, and the loss of family members and friends. This said, very few studies have been performed that look at the relation between war experience and children and adolescents' aggressive behaviours. This study investigated the post traumatic issues of Lebanese adolescents after the war in 2006 and its relation to resiliency and internalising and externalising aggressive behaviours in a sample of 549 Lebanese adolescents from four main regions in Lebanon: Beirut, South Lebanon, Bekaa Valley, and North Lebanon. Resiliency was found to mediate between war traumas and internalising behaviours in a sample of Lebanese adolescents from the South Lebanon and the Bekaa Valley. More specifically, emotional reactivity was found to mediate the relation between shelling and internalising behaviour in a sample of Lebanese adolescents from the South of Lebanon, whereas sense of relatedness was found to mediate the relation between involvement in hostilities and internalising behaviours in a sample of Lebanese adolescents from the Bekaa Valley.

Keywords

adolescents – externalising behaviours – internalising behaviours – Lebanon – resiliency – war

1 Introduction

Research around the impact of armed conflict on children and adolescents' psychological state has increased in recent years[1] yet the issue is still minimally

1 William Yule et al., 'The Long-Term Psychological Effects of a Disaster Experienced in Adolescence: I: The Incidence and Course of PTSD,' *Journal of Child Psychology and Psychiatry*

 | DOI:10.1163/9789004397576_006

addressed. Adolescents in conflict settings are a voiceless population whose needs are often disregarded as they are considered minor compared to the needs of the soldiers and the necessities of war. Children and adolescents have been murdered, raped, and exposed to all sorts of brutality.[2] In the past two decades, approximately two million children have been killed during war and six million injured.[3] Of war survivors, one million children and adolescents have lost both parents[4] and 1.6 million Syrian children were displaced to refugee camps since 2012.[5]

During the Lebanese and Israeli war of July 2006, Lebanese adolescents have been exposed to a large number of traumatic events such as shelling, displacement, witnessing violence, injuries, and the loss of family members and friends.[6] According to a report by the International Committee of the Red Cross, children and adolescents are often exposed to risks associated with war and armed conflicts more than adults;[7] for example, 75 per cent of injuries incurred from landmines in Somalia were to children and adolescents aged between five and fifteen years.[8] Despite all of the foregoing, adolescents still rarely receive the attention and assistance needed to cope with such traumatic experiences both during and after war.

Very few studies have been performed that explicitly examine the relation between war experience and children's and adolescents' aggressive behaviours. Children and adolescents who have experienced war are sometimes described as aggressive and revengeful. However, evidence supporting the claim about aggressiveness among war-traumatised adolescents is sparse and contradictory. The argument that the human mind is a reflection of outside reality and

---

41.4 (2000): 506; Brian K. Barber, 'Making Sense and No Sense of War: Issues of Identity and Meaning in Adolescents' Experience with Political Conflict,' *Adolescents and War: How Youth Deal with Political Violence*, ed. Brian K. Barber (New York: Oxford University Press, 2008).

2 Graca Machel, 'For the Sake of Our Children,' *World Today* 57 (2001): 5.

3 Elisabeth Rasmusson, 'Safeguarding the Children,' *Perspective: Humanitarian and International Affairs Magazine*, April 2011, 6–7.

4 Carol Bellamy, *The State of the World's Children 2002: Leadership* (New York: United Nations Children's Fund, 2002).

5 United Nations High Commissioner for Refugees, 'Syria Regional Refugee Response,' *UNHCR.org*, 2014, viewed 15 May 2016, http://data.unhcr.org/syrianrefugees/regional.php.

6 Rana Tayara, 'Resiliency and War Experiences: A Psychometric Study of the Lebanese Adolescent Experience of War,' *International Journal of Psychology and Behavioral Sciences* 3 (2013): 25.

7 International Committee of the Red Cross, 'Children and War,' ICRC.org, viewed 15 May 2016, https://www.icrc.org/eng/assets/files/other/icrc_002_0577k_children_in_war_kit.pdf.

8 Ibid.

therefore, when you live with violence, you become violent yourself, is not valid in child development. On the contrary, environmental experiences are mediated through cultural symbols,[9] personality, and the coping capacity of the person having the experiences.[10] One should also take into consideration that, in life endangering situations such as war and military violence, several moderating factors related to the child's family and community protect mental health and may explain differences in children and youths' susceptibility to traumatic events.[11]

Finally, the view that war violence produces individual aggression is based on the notion or idea that desire for revenge and feelings of animosity determine how victims will respond. However, alternative responses are also possible as shown by the Japanese Hibakusha group and the South African Truth and Reconciliation committee. Similarly, Barber[12] showed that adolescents' meaning–making experiences of war differed considerably between youths interviewed in Bosnia and the Palestinian youths who had been involved in the Jewish/Arab conflict, where the Palestinians considered that they were helping to make history whilst the dominant view of the Bosnian youths was that they had lost their childhood. Therefore, for the Palestinians, it could be argued that the conflict had enhanced their sense of mastery and therefore their sense of competence and self-efficacy, despite being politically weaker, as is popularly portrayed in the media through news items showing children and adolescents throwing stones and acting aggressively towards the opposition. The Lebanese community has also expressed concern about children's aggressive behaviour as an effect of living in war zones. The first question to be asked is, whether aggressive responses are more common among Lebanese adolescents living in the Bekaa Valley who, during the July 2006 war, were exposed to more severe war experiences than their peers living in the North of Lebanon? The second question is, whether resiliency can protect war exposed adolescents from developing internalised or externalised behaviours?

In simple words, resilience explains why some children overcome seemingly overwhelming obstacles while others become victims of their experiences. In the last fifty years, longitudinal studies of youth facing adversity have found that some that turn up to be resilient do not just recover from the adversity, but they

9 Lev S. Vygotsky, *Mind in Society* (Cambridge, MA: Harvard University Press, 1978).

10 Richard S. Lazarus, 'Coping Theory and Research: Past, Present, and Future,' *Psychosomatic Medicine* 55.3 (1993): 237.

11 Raija-Leena Punamaki, et al., 'The Role of Psychological Defences in Moderating between Trauma and Post-Traumatic Symptoms among Palestinian Men,' *International Journal of Psychology* 37.5 (2002): 289.

12 Barber, 'Making Sense and No Sense of War.'

even manage to thrive. They are those who are able to deal with stress while coping with everyday challenges as well as adversity and traumatic events. Resilient youth appear capable of developing clear and realistic goals, solving problems, relating comfortably with others and treating themselves and others with respect.[13]

Lebanon has been in wars since 1948, after the declaration of the Israeli state on the southern border of Lebanon, and the flooding of around 100,000 Palestinian refugees into Lebanese territories. On the other hand the Palestine Liberation Organization (PLO) went on to recruit militants in Lebanon and started to conduct raids into Israel from Lebanese territories. This led Israel to start retaliatory raids against Lebanese villages. This sparked an arms race between the Lebanese political factions who were pro the PLO and those who were against and provided the start of the Lebanese Civil War that lasted from 1975 till 1990. The 14-year conflict left as many as 200,000 dead and up to a million displaced, internally and internationally. Many Lebanese cities were left in ruins as a result of the bombardments.[14] Israel took advantage of the Civil War and in 1982 it invaded again the Lebanese territories and laid siege to Beirut. In 1983, the United States brokered the May 17 Agreement, a peace treaty between Israel and Lebanon in all but name. Though the majority of the Lebanese civil war conflicts ended beginning of 1990, Israel kept maintaining a military presence in South Lebanon. Furthermore, combat between Israeli forces and Hezbollah (a Lebanese political and religious party) forces kept on going leading to the Operation Grapes of Wrath which resulted in the deaths of more than 150 civilians and refugees, most of them in the shelling of a United Nations base at Qana, South Lebanon. The ongoing hostilities came to an initial end by June 2000 with the withdrawal of Israel from the Lebanese territories.[15]

Unfortunately the combat started once more when on 12 July 2006, militants from Hezbollah fired rockets at Israeli border towns as a diversion for an anti-tank missile attack on two armoured Humvees patrolling the Israeli side of the border fence. The ambush left three soldiers dead. Two Israeli soldiers were abducted and taken by Hezbollah to Lebanon. Five more were killed in Lebanon, in a failed rescue attempt. Hezbollah demanded the release of Lebanese prisoners held by Israel in exchange for the release of the abducted

13 David Murphey et al., 'Positive Mental Health: Resilience,' *Child Trends* 3 (2013): 2.

14 United Nations – General Assembly, 'Implementation of General Assembly Resolution 60/251 of 15 March 2006 Entitled "Human Rights Council": Opinions adopted by the Working Group on Arbitrary Detention,' 2 February 2007, RefWorld.org, viewed 15 May 2016, http://www.refworld.org/docid/470b77b40.html.

15 UN Commission on Human Rights, 'Question of the Violation of Human Rights in the Occupied Arab Territories, including Palestine,' 12 August 2004, A/59/256, viewed 15 May 2016, http://www.refworld.org/docid/4267b5d14.html.

soldiers. Israel refused and responded with airstrikes and artillery fire on targets in Lebanon. Israel attacked both Hezbollah military targets and Lebanese civilian infrastructure, including Beirut's Rafic Hariri International Airport. The Israel Defence Forces (IDF) launched a ground invasion of southern Lebanon. Israel also imposed an air and naval blockade. Hezbollah then launched more rockets into northern Israel and engaged the IDF in guerrilla warfare from hardened positions.[16]

The conflict is believed to have killed between 1191 and 1300 Lebanese people, and 165 Israelis. It severely damaged Lebanese civil infrastructure, and displaced approximately one million Lebanese and 300,000–500,000 Israelis. In this war, Lebanese adolescents have been the targets of killing, beatings and many other forms of violence.[17]

Fortunately, there has been some variation in the intensity of the war between the different regions in Lebanon as not all cities were affected equally, mostly due to their geographical location. North Lebanon, the least affected area, lies 204 km from Haifa. South Lebanon and the Bekaa Valley, two of the most affected areas, lie 55 km and 100 km respectively. Furthermore, The South of Lebanon and the Bekaa Valley were Israel's main target along with the South of Beirut as these three regions are considered as Hezbollah's main quarter. People residing in the North Lebanon and Bekaa Valley therefore differ in their exposure to levels of war experience and destruction. This break in combat has allowed for the examination of war experience as a risk factor for aggressive behaviour in those two Lebanese areas (North Lebanon and the Bekaa Valley).

Recently, researchers in the field of developmental psychology have given much attention to children and adolescents' externalising and internalising behavioural problems.[18] Internalizing behaviour comes with anxiety, depression, and withdrawal from others. Externalizing behaviour consists of a child acting out with aggression, violence, harassment, disruptiveness, and defiance.[19]

---

16 Lebanon Higher Relief Council, 'Lebanon under Siege,' Page archived by TheWaybackMachine.org, viewed 15 May 2016, http://archive.org/web/web.php.

17 Mona S. Macksoud and J. Lawrence Aber, 'The War Experiences and Psychosocial Development of Children in Lebanon,' *Child Development* 67.1 (1996): 75; Tayara, 'Resiliency and War Experiences,' 30.

18 Thomas M. Achenbach and Leslie A. Rescorla, *Manual for the ASEBA School Age Forms and Profiles* (Burlington VT: University of Vermont, Research Center for Children, Youth and Families, 2001).

19 Liu Jianghong, 'Childhood Externalizing Behavior: Theory and Implications,' *Journal of Child Adolescent Psychiatry Nurse* 17.3 (2004): 93–103.

Research has shown that externalising problems are associated with and predicting school failure and juvenile delinquency among other problems.[20] In contrast, adolescents with internalising behavioural problems tend to have maladaptive emotional outcomes such as negative self-perception and depression.[21] According to Rubin and his colleagues, adolescents who display externalising or internalising behaviours are likely to be disliked or rejected by their peers.[22] Externalising and internalising behaviours are simply a reaction from adolescents to their stress experiences. There is also evidence in the literature that adequate coping skills and resilience could prevent aggression among adolescents living in war context and violent communities.[23] Yet there are still significant gaps in the knowledge about the factors associated with resilient outcomes in war- affected adolescents, creating a need to examine more deeply resiliency in war- affected adolescents.

This study looks at the relationship between war experience and externalising and internalising behaviours in four sets of data drawn from Lebanese adolescents. The areas studied are first divided by different degrees of shelling, separation, bereavement, experiencing combat and witnessing violence. Secondly, the current research looks at studying the role of resiliency as a mediator between war experiences and behavioural problems, as measured by the Youth Self Report,[24] in the sample of Lebanese adolescents from the Bekaa Valley. The individuals, in the Bekaa Valley, were the most affected by severe war related experiences.

The hypotheses of the current study states first, a difference might be expected between adolescents from areas severely exposed to war experiences and those from areas less exposed in regards to internalising and externalising behaviour. There is no clear yet direction that the effect is predicted to fall. Second,

20 Achenbach and Rescorla, *Manual for the ASEBA School Age Forms and Profiles*; Kenneth H. Rubin et al., 'The Waterloo Longitudinal Project: Predicting Internalizing and Externalizing Problems in Adolescence,' *Development and Psychopathology* 7 (1995): 755.

21 Michel Boivin, Shelley Hymel and William M. Bukowski, 'The Roles of Social Withdrawal, Peer Rejection, and Victimization by Peers in Predicting Loneliness and Depressed Mood in Childhood,' *Development and Psychopathology* 7 (1995): 770.

22 Kenneth H. Rubin, William M. Bukowski and Jefferey Parker, 'Peer Interactions, Relationships, and Groups,' *Handbook of Child Psychology: Vol. 3 Social, Emotional and Personality Development*, ed. William. E. Damon (New York: Wiley, 1998).

23 Muhammad M. Haj-Yahia and Rula Abdo-Kaloti, 'The Rates and Correlates of the Exposure of Palestinian Adolescents to Family Violence: Toward an Integrative-Holistic Approach,' *Child Abuse and Neglect* 27 (2003): 786; Mary J. Rogers and Grayson N. Holmbeck. 'Effects of Inter-Parental Aggression on Children's Adjustment: The Moderating Role of Cognitive Appraisal and Coping,' *Journal of Family Psychology* 11.1 (1997): 127.

24 Achenbach and Rescorla, *Manual for the ASEBA School Age Forms and Profiles*.

it will examine whether resiliency plays a mediator role, in reference to severe war experiences and aggression; it will also explore, if adolescents reporting high resiliency are less aggressive and cope with life stressors in a better manner.

2 Study I: Internalising and Externalising Behaviours in Lebanese Adolescents Post-War

2.1 *Participants*

The participants for Study I comprised a convenient sample of 549 Lebanese adolescents from Beirut (n = 149; M = 14.71 years, SD = 1.73), South Lebanon (n = 140; M = 15.35 years, SD = 1.24), North Lebanon (n = 124; M = 14.84 years, SD = 1.32) and the Bekaa Valley (n = 136; M = 14.99 years, SD = 1.13). The sample comprised of 277 males and 272 females. The participants were from schools around Lebanon that accepted to take part in the study. Unfortunately, some schools had their reservation regarding allowing their students to participate out of concern and fear, regardless of the anonymity of the questionnaires.

2.2 *Procedure*

All necessary approvals were obtained prior to commencement of the study in June 2007 almost a year after the 2006 war. The collection of the data ended in August 2007. Participants completed both the Youth Self Report and the War Experience Survey. Study participants were informed that there were no right or wrong answers and that their honesty in responding to the scales was an important factor for the study.

2.3 *Measurements*

The Youth Self Report (YSR) is derived from the Child Behaviour Checklist (CBCL) and designed for use with adolescents between the ages of 12 and 18. The YSR contains two sub-areas, the first being twenty competence items measuring the adolescents' participation in different activities including sports, chores, jobs, games, friends and hobbies. The second sub-area contains 112 Likert scale items from 0 (not true) to 2 (very or often true) measuring eight sub-scale symptoms: withdrawal, somatic complaints, anxiety and depression, social problems, thought problems, attention problems, aggressive behaviours and delinquent behaviours. Subscales include items such as: 'I refuse to talk'; 'I don't have much energy'; 'I physically attack people'; 'I break rules at home, school or elsewhere.'[25]

25 Ibid.

The first three subscales (withdrawn, somatic complaints and anxiety and depression) are summed to form the internalising behaviours subscale and the last two subscales (aggressive behaviours and delinquent behaviours) are thought to form the externalising behaviours subscale. The remaining three subscales (social, thought and attention problems) are not categorised as internalising or externalising and should be looked at separately. For the purpose of this current study, the last three subscales are thought to be irrelevant and were not included in the analyses. The problem scale total is thought to provide a measurement of the overall behavioural and emotional functioning of the adolescents.

Although the YSR had been translated to Arabic prior to this study, no normative data from Lebanon are available.[26] A reliability measurement (a measurement that indicates the degree of internal consistency where items in the surveys used are measured for relatedness and variability) was performed for this study's sample and was found to be satisfactory (alpha = .94). The coefficients were modest when investigated by the individual subscales and by gender; they varied between .52 (anxious-depressed) and .88 (externalising-behaviours). These coefficients were not dissimilar to those reported by Achenbach[27] except for the anxious-depressed subscale, the withdrawn-depressed subscale and the attention problems subscale.

The moderate intercorrelation of the Arabic YSR scales provides support for the multidimensionality of the measure in Lebanese adolescents. In the current study the overall goal of the YSR was to classify respondents' answers as either internalising or externalising behaviours and, therefore, only data on the second sub-area of the YSR is discussed.

The War Experience Survey is a short survey that includes ten war trauma categories created by Macksoud and Aber.[28] The War Experience Survey is rated on a 3-point Likert scale scored as mildly affected, affected, and extremely affected. The ten war trauma items form three subscales: active involvement, passive involvement, and loss.[29]

2.4 *Results*

Nonparametric tests were used in the current study because these tests are considered more capable than parametric tests of detecting population differences when certain assumptions (such as test of homogeneity) are not satisfied. Gender and age differences were first reported using a series of

26 Ibid.

27 Ibid.

28 Macksoud and Aber, 'The War Experiences and Psychosocial Development,' 78.

29 Tayara, 'Resiliency and War Experiences,' 29.

Mann-Whitney tests. Furthermore, in order to examine regional differences for internalising and externalising behaviours data given by the Youth Self Report, a Kruskal-Wallis test was first computed, (because the data being analysed are data gathered from four different populations and assumed to not be identical without assuming the normal distribution). This was followed by a series of Mann-Whitney tests. A Spearman's correlation test was also conducted to explore the strength of relationships between war experiences data (as reported by the WES), and internalising and externalising behaviour data (as reported by the YSR).

Mann-Whitney tests were conducted to evaluate pairwise differences between age and gender on internalising behaviours, controlling for any Type I error across tests using the Bonferroni approach. The results of these tests indicated no significant difference between males and females on internalising behaviours U (17) = 9193 value, Z = -.25, p = .80. On the other hand, a significant difference was perceived between males and females on externalising behaviours U (18) = 8086 value Z = -2.13, p = .03. The mean of externalising behaviours among male adolescents was higher than among female adolescents.

As for age differences, Mann-Whitney tests indicated significant difference between young adolescents (between 13 and 15 years of age) older adolescents (between 16 and 18 years of age) in regards to internalising behaviours U (14) = 8264 value Z = -1.13, p = .02. No such difference has been found in regards to externalising behaviours.

The internalising and externalising behaviours found in Lebanon were analysed. The Kruskal-Wallis test was computed to examine differences between the four regions in internalising behaviours data and externalising behaviours data. The results of the analysis indicates that there is a significant difference between the medians of internalising behaviours data for the groups, $x^2(3, N = 549) = 8.23, p = .04$. The proportion of variability in the ranked dependent variable accounted for by the regions was 45.18 indicating a fairly strong relationship between regions and internalising behaviours. No such significance existed in the medians of externalising behaviours data $x^2(3, N = 549) = 5.04, p = .17$. Table 4.3 shows the different mean rank of internalising behaviours data and externalising behaviours data according to the four different regions.

Follow-up Mann-Whitney tests were conducted to evaluate pairwise differences among the four regions on internalising behaviours data. The results of these tests indicated a significant difference between the Bekaa Valley group and the North of Lebanon group U (3) = 7722 value, Z = -2.34, *p* = .02.

The mean of internalising behaviours data among adolescents in the Bekaa Valley was lower than among adolescents in the North Lebanon. A significant

TABLE 4.1 Gender differences for externalising and internalising behaviours

		N	Mean	Std. deviation
Internalising	Male	278	15.42	7.05
	Female	271	16.17	6.60
Externalising	Male	278	18.30	10.06
	Female	271	16.78	9.85

TABLE 4.2 Age differences for externalising and internalising behaviours (N = 549)

		N	Mean	Std. dev.
Internalising	16–18 years	310	15.50	6.50
	13–15 years	239	16.18	7.23
Externalising	16–18 years	310	17.14	9.78
	13–15 years	239	18.08	10.24

TABLE 4.3 Mean rank of internalising and externalising behaviours by regions

Living areas		N	Mean rank
Internalising	Beirut	149	287
	South of Lebanon	140	255
	North of Lebanon	124	300
	Bekaa Valley	136	256
Externalising	Beirut	149	293
	South of Lebanon	140	258
	North of Lebanon	124	285
	Bekaa Valley	136	261

difference also existed between the South Lebanon and the North Lebanon group U (3) = 7247 value, Z = -2.14, p =.03. No differences were found between Beirut and any of the other three regions.

The differences found in the mean of internalising behaviours between adolescents in South Lebanon, Bekaa Valley and North Lebanon may be due to war experiences. In order to further examine this result, the relation between internalising and externalising behaviours data and war experience data was investigated.

The correlation between internalising and externalising behaviours data and war experience data, controlling for age and gender was analysed using a Spearman's correlation test, that revealed that internalising behaviours data were negatively correlated with reported total war experience in the Bekaa Valley ($r = -.18$; $p<.05$) and the South Lebanon ($r = -11$, $p<.05$), while externalising behaviours data had no significant correlations with reported war experience in any of the four regions studied (Table 4.4).

2.5 *Discussion*

The reliability (in terms of internal consistency among the measurement items in a given survey) of the Arabic version of the YSR used on a sample of 549 Lebanese adolescents was found to be satisfactory (alpha = .94). The positive intercorrelations between anxious-depressed data, withdrawn-depressed data and somatic complaints data are not surprising as they all measure the same construct of internalising behaviours. This positive intercorrelation was also found between rule breaking behaviours data and aggressive behaviours data that also measure one higher order construct, externalised behaviours.

Gender differences were found in regard to externalising behaviours data as males reported higher rates of externalising ($M = 18.30$, $SD = 10.06$) behaviours than females ($M = 16.78$, $SD = 9.85$). These results correspond with previous research[30] as although both females and males suffering from trauma could end up suffering from behavioural problems, the literature suggests a significant distinction between boys and girls coping responses.[31] Literature has shown that males can, may react to stress differently than females as they often cope with stress by externalising their behaviour, a coping mechanism that some females tend to avoid. Therefore, when confronted with stress or traumatic experiences, boys may have a higher tendency than girls to express anger and act out aggressively, although Lebanese boys were just as likely to experience internalising behaviour as girls

30 Timothy O. Ireland, Carolyn A. Smith, and Terence B. Thornberry, 'Developmental Issues in the Impact of Child Maltreatment on Later Delinquency and Drug Use,' *Criminology* 40.2 (2002): 375; Heike Eschenbeck, Carl W. Kohlman and Arnold Lohaus, 'Gender Differences in Coping Strategies in Children and Adolescents,' *Journal of Individual Differences* 28.1 (2007): 23.

31 Eschenbeck et al., 'Gender Differences,' 24.

TABLE 4.4 Relation between internalising and externalising behaviours and war

	Internalising	Externalising	War experience
Beirut			
Internalising	1.00	.63**	.04
Externalising		1.00	.12
War Experience			1.00
South of Lebanon			
Internalising	1.00	.62**	-.11*
Externalising		1.00	-.04
War Experience			1.00
North of Lebanon			
Internalising	1.00	.66**	.30
Externalising		1.00	.08
War Experience			1.00
Bekaa Valley			
Internalising	1.00	.56**	-.18*
Externalising		1.00	-.13
War Experience			1.00

* P < 0.05; ** P <0.01

in this study. This is in contrast to the wider pool of literature that suggests that females are more likely to cope with stress and trauma by internalising their behaviours.[32]

In order to study the differences in internalising and externalising behaviours data amongst the four regions of Lebanon taking part in the current study, a Kruskal-Wallis test was computed and found that such significance only exists in regard to internalising behaviours. A Mann-Whitney test was conducted to evaluate pairwise differences amongst the four regions for internalising behaviours data. A significance difference was found between the two samples of adolescents from the Bekaa Valley, and South Lebanon and the sample of adolescents from the North of Lebanon. This difference may be due to the relation between internalising behaviour and the exposure to traumatic experiences. Data suggests that adolescents from Bekaa Valley and the

32 Ireland et al., 'Developmental Issues.'

South of Lebanon were exposed to a higher number of war experiences, as well as to more severe types of war experiences, than adolescents from the North of Lebanon. A Spearman's correlation test was conducted that found internalising behaviours data had a negative correlation with reported war experiences data among adolescents in the Bekaa Valley. Interaction effects between age, gender and war experiences on externalising and internalising behaviour were non-significant, indicating that the relationship between the witnessing of war experiences and adolescents' aggression was present for all ages and gender. These findings confirm the stated hypothesis as a difference was found between data gathered from adolescents from areas of severe exposure to war and those from areas less exposed in regard to internalising and externalising data.

This relation between war experience data and externalising and internalising behaviour data could be moderated by other variables such as resiliency, as the Lebanese adolescent data had revealed meaningful patterns of correlations in regard to resiliency and war experiences. According to a previous finding by Tayara, adolescents who witnessed violence or were injured were more likely to report a higher sense of mastery and a lower sense of emotional reactivity.[33] Emotional reactivity measures negative resiliency, while a sense of mastery and sense of relatedness are scored in a positive direction. In contrast, adolescents who suffered the loss of a relative or a friend through separation or bereavement, reported a lower sense of mastery and relatedness due to their loss.[34] Similar findings have been made in previous research, where resilient adolescents were reported to be more capable of coping with the stress that comes with experiencing armed conflicts and war.[35]

The second study reported below, looks at the relationship between internalising behaviours data and war experiences data as mediated by resiliency data in the South of Lebanon and the Bekaa Valley. These two regions of Lebanon have been selected as adolescents located here reported lower rates on internalising behaviours data than their peers in Beirut and North Lebanon and experienced a greater level of conflict than those in Beirut and North Lebanon.

33 Tayara, 'Resiliency and War Experiences,' 30.

34 Ibid.

35 Stephen Joseph, P. Alex Linley, and George J. Harris, 'Understanding Positive Change Following Trauma and Adversity: Structural Clarification,' *Journal of Loss and Trauma* 10 (2005): 86.

3 Study II: The Mediation Effect of Resiliency in Internalising and Externalising Behaviour

3.1 *Participants*

The participants for Study II comprised the same sample of 276 Lebanese adolescents from South of Lebanon (n = 140, *M* = 15.35, *SD* = 1.24), and the Bekaa Valley (n = 136, *M* = 14.99, *SD* = 1.13) reported in Study I.

3.2 *Measurements*

The Resiliency Scale for Children and Adolescents- Arabic (RSCA) is a self-report questionnaire that measures three areas of perceived strength and/or vulnerability related to psychological resilience, according to Sandra Prince-Embury, with response options rated on a 5 point Likert scale ranging from 0 (Never) to 5 (Almost Always).[36] The scales include two positive factors sense of mastery, a sense of relatedness; and one negative, emotional reactivity. Sense of mastery as defined by Embury, represents youths' self-perceptions of their skills and competence. The sense of mastery subscale includes items such as: 'If I try hard, it makes a difference'; 'I can let others help me when I need to.' Sense of relatedness refers to youths' perceived quality of their relationships. Sense of relatedness includes items such as: 'I can make up with friends after a fight'; 'if something bad happens, I can ask my parent(s) for help.' The last subscale refers to negative resilience and is known as emotional reactivity. Emotional reactivity assesses how well youth feel about being able to control their emotions. Youth with high emotional reactivity have difficulties controlling their emotions. Items on the emotional reactivity subscales include: 'I can make up with friends after a fight'; 'If something bad happens, I can ask my parent(s) for help.' The Arab-language version was created, adapted, and validated by Tayara.[37]

3.3 *Results*

A series of regression analyses were performed to examine the role of resiliency as a mediator variable with the war experience sub-scales as predictors of internalising behaviour. An analysis of items was undertaken to provide further clarification and two models were generated to understand the relation between specific war experiences data, resiliency subscales data and behavioural

36 Sandra Prince-Embury, *Resiliency Scales for Adolescents: Profiles of Personal Strengths* (San Antonio, TX: Harcourt Assessments, 2006).

37 Tayara, 'Resiliency and War Experiences,' 29.

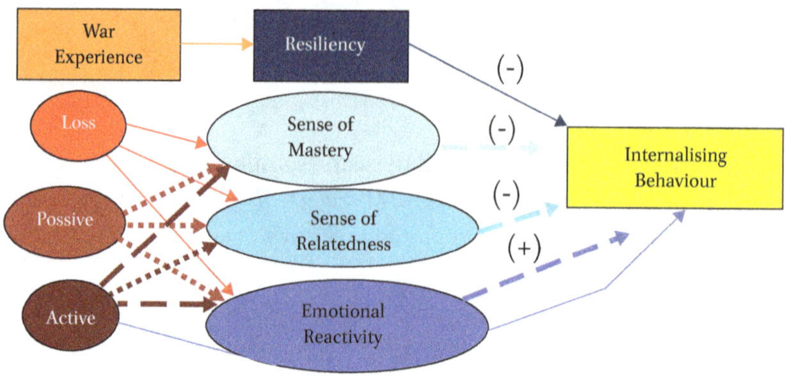

FIGURE 4.1 Model depicting the relation between war experience and internalising behaviour as mediated by resiliency

outcomes data. The war experience items, and war experiences subscales with the highest variance were chosen for further investigation.

In accordance with Baron and Kenny, the prerequisites for a mediation model are a relationship between the predictor and outcome variables.[38] In this study, these factors are: resiliency, war experience and internalising behaviour. To test the hypothesis that resiliency is a mediator between war experiences and aggression, a series of regression analyses were carried out for each of the two regions separately. In this case a model was developed with the war experience subscales (loss, passive involvement, active involvement) as the predictor variables, the resiliency subscales (sense of mastery, sense of relatedness, emotional reactivity) applied separately as the mediator variable and internalising behaviour as the outcome variable.

It must be shown that the predictor significantly predicts the outcome. As such, a regression analysis was performed with the different war experiences entered as the predictor and scores on internalising behaviour data as the outcome variable. The predictor must be significant predictor of the mediator variable. As such, the different war experiences were entered into the regression analyses with the resiliency subscale scores as the outcome variable. The mediator must be shown to still be significantly related to the outcome variable when controlling for the variance with the predictor. As such, the WES scores and the resiliency scores were entered into a regression analysis with internalising behaviour as the outcome. If the relationship between the

38 Reuben M. Baron and David A. Kenny, 'The Moderator-Mediator Variable Distinction in Social Psychological Research: Conceptual, Strategic, and Statistical Considerations,' *Journal of Personality and Social Psychology* 51.6 (1986): 1175.

predictor and the outcome is zero once the mediator is controlled for then it is a complete mediator. If the regression coefficient is only reduced then it is a partial mediator. Figure 4.1 depicts a model describing the pathway of war experience to internalised behaviour as mediated by resiliency.

War experience data was shown to correlate negatively with internalising behaviour data in a sample of Lebanese adolescents from the Bekaa Valley (N=136), and a sample of Lebanese adolescents from the South of Lebanon (N=140). In order to further understand the relation between internalising behaviour data, multiple regression analysis has been performed by entering the ten different war experiences as predictors and scores on internalising behaviour data as outcome with a sample of 276 Lebanese adolescents controlling for age, gender, and religion. The results indicated that although loss, active involvement, and passive involvement did not significantly account for the variance in internalising behaviour data, shelling experience data was negatively related to internalising behaviour data (beta= -1.46, $p < .05$) in adolescents in the South (Table 4.5).

Furthermore, data for involvement in hostilities was positively related to internalised behaviour data (beta = 1.58, $p < .05$) in adolescents from the Bekaa Valley (Table 4.6). Therefore, shelling data will be further investigated as a possible predictor of lower internalised behaviour data scores in adolescents living in the South of Lebanon. In contrast, data scores for involvement in hostilities will be studied further as a possible predictor of internalised behaviour scores in adolescents from the Bekaa Valley.

This author studied the relation between war experiences and resiliency subscales in a sample of 549 Lebanese adolescents from four regions (Beirut, South Lebanon, North Lebanon and the Bekaa Valley) and found that for the whole sample, witnessing violence scores predicted a higher sense of mastery scores while bereavement scores predicted a lower sense of mastery scores. Furthermore, data on being injured predicted higher emotional reactivity scores while displacement scores predicted a low sense of relatedness scores.[39] For the current study, similar analyses were conducted for the sample of 276 Lebanese from the South of Lebanon and the Bekaa Valley.

The analyses showed that in regard to the sample from the South of Lebanon, for sense of mastery, loss accounted for 6% of the variance, passive involvement accounted for 5% of the variance, and finally active involvement accounted for 5.5% of the variance. More specifically, deprivation experience data (beta = -.34, SE = .15, $p < .02$), and taking part in combat data (beta = -.22,

39 Tayara, 'Resiliency and War Experiences,' 30.

TABLE 4.5 Relationship between war traumas and internalising behaviour in the south

Variables	Internalising behaviour		
	Beta	SE	Sig
Demographics			
Age	-.96*	.50	0.5
Gender	.07	1.23	.95
Religion	.29	1.18	.80
R^2	.03	7.07	
$F(3, 137)$	1.23		.30
Loss			
Bereavement	-.11	.70	.88
Displacement	1.34	1.55	.39
Separation	-1.37	1.97	.49
Emigration	-.76	1.08	.48
R^2	.04	7.13	
$F(6, 134)$	.76		.61
Passive Involvement			
Deprivation	-3.32	2.96	.26
Shelling	**-1.46***	**.81**	**.04**
Witnessing Violence	1.81	1.55	.24
R^2	.04	7.04	
$F(6,134)$	1.64		
Active Involvement			
Injuries	.09	.97	.93
Involvement in Hostilities	1.76	3.72	.64
Combat	1.44	2.03	.48
R^2	.03	7.13	
$F(6, 134)$	.75		.60

* $p < 0.05$; ** $p < 0.01$

SE = .05, p < .03) were found to be negatively related to sense of mastery data. Whereas separation data (beta = .25, SE = .05, p < .01) was found to be positively related to sense of mastery data (Table 4.7).

For the sense of relatedness scoring, loss accounted for 13%, passive involvement for 14% and finally active involvement for 9% of the variance for south of

TABLE 4.6 Relationship between war traumas scores and internalising behaviour scores in Bekaa Valley

Variables	Internalising behaviour		
	Beta	**SE**	**Sig**
Demographics			
Age	.48	.54	.37
Gender	1.49	1.21	.22
Religion	.230	.97	.81
R^2	.02	6.87	
$F(3, 132)$	.66		.58
Loss			
Bereavement	.82	.86	.34
Displacement	-.81	.65	.21
Separation	-.35	.70	.62
Emigration	2.04	1.35	.13
R^2	.06	6.83	
$F(6, 129)$	1.07		3.85
Passive Involvement			
Deprivation	.82	1.09	.45
Shelling	.40	.86	.64
Witnessing Violence	-.91	.80	.25
R^2	.03	6.90	
$F(4, 131)$	.60		.73
Active Involvement			
Injuries	.32	1.14	.78
Involvement in Hostilities	**1.58***	**.95**	**.05**
Combat	.27	.59	64
R^2	.04	6.86	
$F(3, 132)$	.85		.53

Lebanon. More specifically, witnessing violence data (beta = .21, SE = .08) and separation data (beta = .11, SE = .06) were positively related to sense of relatedness scores, while deprivation data (beta = -.39, SE = .16) was negatively related to sense of relatedness scores (Table 4.8).

Finally, for emotional reactivity within the south of Lebanon group; loss accounted for 23%, and passive involvement for 14% of the variance, while active

TABLE 4.7 Relationship between war traumas and sense of mastery in the south

Variables	Sense of mastery		
	Beta	SE	Sig
Age	.00	.02	.95
Gender	-.07	.06	.27
Religion	-.04	.06	.56
R^2	.01	.36	
F(3, 136)	.47		.70
Loss			
Bereavement	-.09	.08	.39
Displacement	-.05	.35	.61
Separation	**.25****	**.05**	**.01**
Emigration	-.02	.09	.88
R^2	.06	.36	
F(7, 132)	**1.24***		**.05**
Passive Involvement			
Deprivation	**-.34***	**.15**	**.02**
Shelling	.40	.86	.64
Witnessing Violence	-.91	.80	.25
R^2	.05	.361	
F(6, 133)	**1.20***		**.05**
Active Involvement			
Injuries	-.02	.18	.89
Involvement in Hostilities	.05	.10	.64
Combat	**-.22***	**.05**	**.03**
R^2	.05	.36	
F(6, 133)	**1.25***		**.05**

involvement did not account for any percentage. Shelling (beta = -.20, SE.05) and displacement (beta = -.23, SE = .05) were negatively related to emotional reactivity. Separation data (beta = .21, SE = .07) was positively related to emotional reactivity.

As for the sample of adolescents from the Bekaa Valley, although none of the total war experiences subscales significantly accounted for the variance

TABLE 4.8 Relationship between war traumas and sense of relatedness in south

Variables	Sense of relatedness		
	Beta	**SE**	**Sig**
Demographics			
Age	-.20	.03	.02
Gender	.22	.07	.01
Religion	.00	.06	.98
R^2	.08	.38	
$F(3, 136)$	.47		.01
Loss			
Bereavement	-.02	.08	.80
Displacement	-.13	.04	.15
Separation	**.11***	**.06**	**.05**
Emigration	.09	.11	.36
R^2	.13	.08	
$F(7, 132)$	**2.74****		**.01**
Passive Involvement			
Deprivation	**-.39****	**.16**	**.01**
Shelling	-.06	.04	.17
Witnessing Violence	**.21****	**.08**	**.01**
R^2	.14	.39	
$F(6, 133)$	**3.52****		**.00**
Active Involvement			
Injuries	.16	.20	.42
Involvement in Hostilities	.05	.11	.63
Combat	-.07	.05	.17
R^2	.09	.38	
$F(6, 133)$	**2.25***		**.05**

found in sense of mastery scores, still scores for witnessing violence on its own (beta = .19, SE = .05, $p < .03$) were positively related to sense of mastery scores (Table 4.10).

For the sense of relatedness scores, only loss accounted for 10% ($p < .01$) of the variance, and more specifically, shelling (beta = -.17, SE = .05, $p < .05$), and displacement (beta = -.20, SE = .04, $p < .01$) were negatively related to sense of relatedness for Bekaa valley subjects. See Table 4.11.

TABLE 4.9 Relationship between war traumas and emotional reactivity in south

Variables	Emotional reactivity		
	Beta	SE	Sig
Demographics			
Age	-.20	.03	.02
Gender	.22	.07	.01
Religion	.00	.06	.98
R^2	.06	.52	
$F(3, 136)$	2.70		.05
Loss			
Bereavement	-.09	.10	.35
Displacement	-.23**	.05	.00
Separation	.21**	.07	.00
Emigration	.16	.13	.21
R^2	.23	.48	
$F(7, 132)$	5.71**		.00
Passive Involvement			
Deprivation	-.11	.21	.58
Shelling	-.20**	.06	.00
Witnessing Violence	.09	.11	.41
R^2	.14	.99	
$F(6, 133)$	3.55**		.00
Active Involvement			
Injuries	.17	.27	.54
Involvement in Hostilities	.09	.15	.52
Combat	-.02	.07	.74
R^2	.06	.02	
$F(3, 136)$	2.70		.20

Finally, for emotional reactivity scores none of the war experience subscales accounted for any of the variance with emotional reactivity for the Bekaa valley participants. In summary, loss, active war experience and passive war experience have been found to partially predict a sense of relatedness and a negative emotional reactivity within the sample of Lebanese adolescents from the South of Lebanon. Whereas only loss has been found to partially predict a sense of relatedness, within the sample of Lebanese adolescents from the Bekaa Valley.

TABLE 4.10 Relationship between war traumas and sense of mastery in the Bekaa

Variables	Sense of mastery		
	Beta	**SE**	**Sig**
Demographics			
Age	.07	.04	.43
Gender	.11	.08	.22
Religion	-.05	.06	.54
R^2	.02	.45	
F(3, 135)	.77		.51
Loss			
Bereavement	-.18	.06	.04
Displacement	-.07	.04	.43
Separation	.02	.05	.83
Emigration	-.06	.09	.50
R^2	.06	.45	
F(7, 135)	1.179		.32
Passive Involvement			
Deprivation	-.12	.07	.19
Shelling	-.08	.05	.30
Witnessing Violence	**.19***	**.05**	**.03**
R^2	-.06	.45	
F(6, 135)	1.36		.24
Active Involvement			
Injuries	-.02	.07	.79
Involvement in Hostilities	.08	.06	.32
Combat	.03	.04	.72
R^2	.03	.46	
F(6, 135)	.58		.74

In order to see whether the relation between war experience data and internalising behaviour data was mediated by resiliency data as stated in our hypothesis, it was important to study once more the relation between war experience data and internalising behaviour data while controlling for the resiliency subscales. According to the previous findings, shelling scores were mainly found to be negatively correlated with internalising behaviour scores in the South, and emotional reactivity scores were found to have a significant negative relation

TABLE 4.11 Relationship between war traumas and sense of relatedness in the Bekaa Valley

Variables	Sense of relatedness		
	Beta	SE	Sig
Demographics			
Age			
Gender			
Religion			
R^2	.02	.45	
$F(3, 135)$	1.76		.16
Loss			
Bereavement	-.12	.06	.18
Displacement	**-.20****	**.04**	**.01**
Separation	.14	.05	.12
Emigration	.14	.09	.76
R^2	.10	.44	
$F(7, 135)$	**1.96***		**.01**
Passive Involvement			
Deprivation	-.08	.07	.36
Shelling	**-.17***	**.05**	**.05**
Witnessing Violence	.09	.05	.33
R^2	.03	.45	
$F(6, 135)$	1.78		.11
Active Involvement			
Injuries	-.03	.07	.71
Involvement in Hostilities	.11	.06	.19
Combat	-.03	.04	.75
R^2	.01	.45	
$F(6, 135)$	1.21		.30

with shelling scores. Therefore, it was of importance to study the role of emotional reactivity as a mediator between shelling and internalising behaviour in the South. Please refer to Figure 4.2. It should be noted that emotional reactivity represents a negative type of resiliency as emotionally reactive adolescents are considered to be more sensitive and more impaired than their peers.[40]

40 Embury, 'Resiliency Scales for Adolescents: Profiles of Personal Strengths.'

TABLE 4.12 Relationship between war traumas and emotional reactivity in the Bekaa Valley

Variables	Emotional reactivity		
	Beta	**SE**	**Sig**
Demographics			
Age	-.01	.04	.91
Gender	.04	.09	.68
Religion	-.12	.07	.18
R^2	.01	.52	
$F(3, 135)$	.76		.52
Loss			
Bereavement	-.13	.06	.16
Displacement	-.01	.05	.87
Separation	-.05	.05	.61
Emigration	-.08	.10	.34
R^2	.05	.52	
$F(7, 135)$	.93		.48
Passive Involvement			
Deprivation	-.03	.08	.72
Shelling	.08	-.05	.60
Witnessing Violence	.06	-.12	.21
R^2	.04	.52	
$F(6, 135)$	.85		.53
Active Involvement			
Injuries	.09	.08	.30
Involvement in Hostilities	.05	.07	.59
Combat	.02	.05	.81
R^2	.03	.52	
$F(6, 135)$	.63		.70

This mediation model was investigated in the sample of adolescents from the South of Lebanon (N = 140, M = 15.35, SD = 1.24). The direct relation between shelling scores and internalising behaviour scores revealed a beta coefficient of -1.46 $p < .01$. When emotional reactivity was studied as the mediator of the model, the relation between shelling (the predictor) and Internalising Behaviour (the outcome) was significantly reduced (beta = .03, $p < .05$) indicating

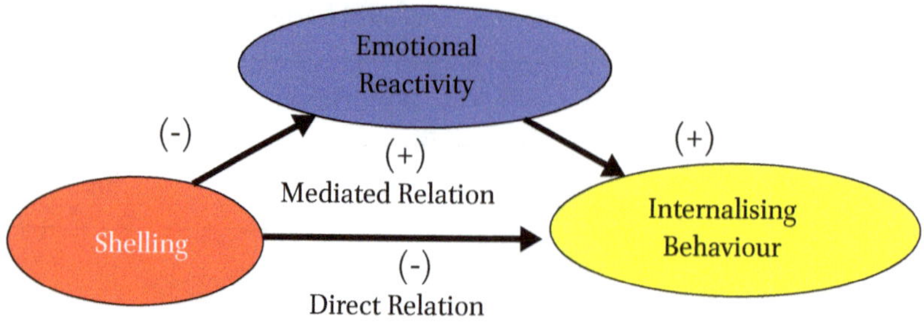

FIGURE 4.2 Model depicting the possible relationship between shelling and internalising behaviour as mediated by emotional reactivity

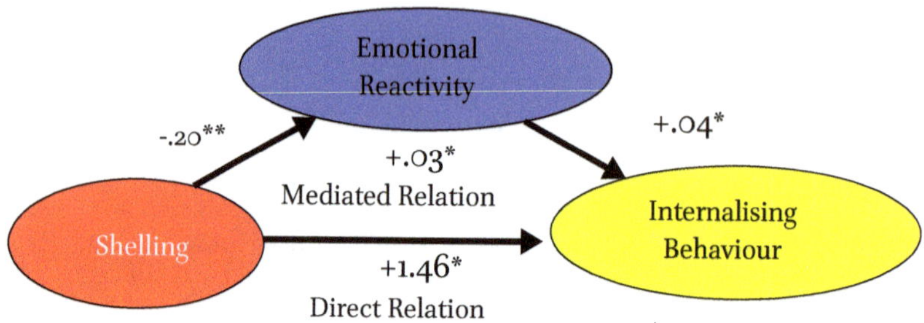

FIGURE 4.3 Model depicting the actual relationship between shelling scores and internalising behaviour scores as mediated by emotional reactivity scores in South Lebanon

that emotional reactivity is a partial mediator between shelling scores and internalising behaviour scores. Although the presence of emotional reactivity as a mediator decreases the relationship between shelling scores and internalised behaviour scores, this relationship turns into a positive one where emotionally reactive adolescents are more likely to be impaired after the trauma and therefore more likely to internalise their aggression. Please see Figure 4.3.

According to the previously mentioned findings of this study, data regarding involvement in hostilities was mainly found to be positively correlated with internalising behaviour scores in the Bekaa Valley, and data regarding sense of relatedness was found to have a significant positive relation with involvement scores for the same sample. Therefore it was of importance to study the role of sense of relatedness as a mediator between involvement in hostilities data and internalising behaviour data in the Bekaa Valley. The role of a sense of relatedness as a mediator for the Bekaa Valley subjects is explored in Figure 4.4.

Within the mediated relation in the sample of adolescents from the Bekaa Valley there was an N of 136, mean of 14.99 years, and a standard

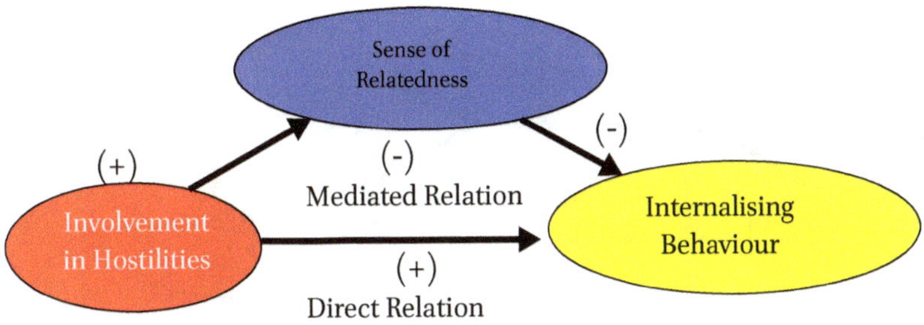

FIGURE 4.4 Model II depicting the predicted relation between involvement in hostilities and internalising behaviour as mediated by sense of relatedness

deviation of 1.13. The direct relationship between involvement in hostilities and internalising behaviour was beta = 1.58, $p < .05$. When the sense of relatedness was looked at as a mediator, the relation between involvement in hostilities (the predictor) and internalising behaviour (the outcome) was significantly reduced (beta = .02, $p < .05$); indicating that a sense of relatedness is a partial mediator between involvement in hostilities and internalising behaviour. Figure 4.5 provides a model of the mediator (sense of relatedness) with the predicator (involvement in hostilities) and the outcome (internalising behaviour).

3.4 *Discussion*

The results of study I among Lebanese adolescents (N = 549) looked at internalising and externalising behaviours in post-war Lebanon. The current study found that although externalising behaviour had no relation with war experiences, internalising behaviours had a negative relationship as reported with an overall total war experience in the Bekaa Valley and the South of Lebanon. One explanation is that being the victim of war and military conflict involves implicit rewards such as heroism and feeling of belonging to a national struggle against foreign occupation. Individuals in such cases receive support, admiration and encouragements from their society, increasing their endurance and therefore their ability to cope with the stress.[41]

Other variables and mediators that play an important role in adolescents coping skills and post war resiliency should be explored. In the current study, shelling seems to result in a lower internalised behaviour and lower emotional

41 Samir Qouta et al., 'Does War Beget Child Aggression? Military Violence, Gender, Age and Aggressive Behavior in Two Palestinian Samples,' *Aggressive Behavior* 34.3 (2008): 235.

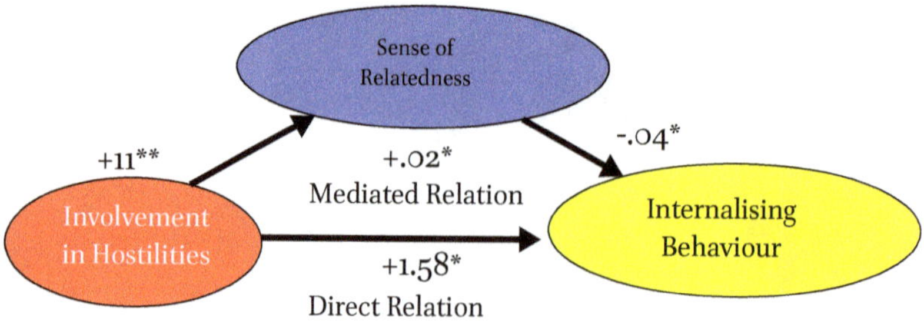

FIGURE 4.5 Model depicting the actual relation between involvement in hostilities and internalising behaviour as mediated by sense of relatedness in the Bekaa Valley

reactivity. Model I found a negative relationship between shelling and internalising behaviour. Emotional reactivity was found to significantly mediate the relation between shelling and internalising behaviour; as adolescents with high emotional reactivity, were unable to cope with shelling and resorted to internalising their aggression.

The results of the current study also found that in the sample of Lebanese adolescents from the Bekaa Valley; involvement in hostilities seemed to predict higher internalised behaviour. Model II explores a sense of relatedness as the mediator between involvement in hostilities and internalising behaviour. It has been found that internalising behaviour and involvement in hostilities are partially mediated by a sense of relatedness. Therefore, adolescents who reported a higher sense of relatedness also report lower internalised behaviour even after being involved in hostilities.

Research has found that some children in similar violent and life threatening environments may become aggressive, while others are more proactive, and show positive coping skills.[42] Our study has identified the differences between the interactions of psychological factors, war experiences and the behaviours that arise from exposure to war, as well as, the possible explanations behind the predictors, behaviours and outcomes. The results found in this study should elevate the importance of planning and establishing not only intervention programs, but also prevention programs, by fostering the concept of resilience early on during elementary schooling and highlighting the importance of well-being (emotional and psychological) in all Arabic countries.

42 Craig A. Anderson and Brad J. Bushman, 'Human Aggression,' *Annual Review of Psychology* 53 (2002): 30.

This said, self-report questionnaires carry methodological problems including inadequate memory, false reports and the desire of the adolescents to be perceived as heroes in the face of severe trauma. However, given the importance of reaching a large number of children from all the main regions in Lebanon, questionnaires were favoured despite their limitations.

Bibliography

Achenbach, Thomas M. and Leslie, A. Rescorla. *Manual for the ASEBA School Age Forms and Profiles.* Burlington VT: University of Vermont, Research Center for Children, Youth and Families, 2001.

Anderson, Craig A. and Brad J. Bushman. 'Human Aggression.' *Annual Review of Psychology* 53 (2002): 27–51.

Barber, Brian K. 'Making Sense and No Sense of War: Issues of Identity and Meaning in Adolescents' Experience with Political Conflict.' *Adolescents and War: How Youth Deal with Political Violence*, edited by Brian K. Barber, 3–32. New York: Oxford University Press, 2008.

Baron, Reuben M. and David A. Kenny. 'The Moderator-Mediator Variable Distinction in Social Psychological Research: Conceptual, Strategic, and Statistical Considerations.' *Journal of Personality and Social Psychology* 51.6 (1986): 1173–1182.

Bellamy, Carol. *The State of the World's Children 2002: Leadership.* New York: United Nations Children's Fund, 2002.

Boivin, Michel, Shelley Hymel and William M. Bukowski. 'The Roles of Social Withdrawal, Peer Rejection, and Victimization by Peers in Predicting Loneliness and Depressed Mood in Childhood.' *Development and Psychopathology* 7 (1995): 765–785.

David Murphey, Megan Barry, and Brigitte Vaughn. 'Positive Mental Health: Resilience.' *Child Trends* 3 (2013): 1–6.

Eschenbeck, Heike, Carl W. Kohlman and Arnold Lohaus. 'Gender Differences in Coping Strategies in Children and Adolescents.' *Journal of Individual Differences* 28.1 (2007): 18–26.

Haj-Yahia, Muhammad M. and Rula Abdo-Kaloti. 'The Rates and Correlates of the Exposure of Palestinian Adolescents to Family Violence: Toward an Integrative-Holistic Approach.' *Child Abuse and Neglect* 27 (2003): 781–806.

International Committee of the Red Cross. 'Children and War.' ICRC.org. Viewed 15 May 2016. https://www.icrc.org/eng/assets/files/other/icrc_002_0577k_children_in_war_kit.pdf.

Ireland, Timothy O., Carolyn A. Smith and Terence B. Thornberry. 'Developmental Issues in the Impact of Child Maltreatment on Later Delinquency and Drug Use.' *Criminology* 40.2 (2002): 359–392.

Jianghong, Liu. 'Childhood Externalizing Behavior: Theory and Implications.' *Journal of Child Adolescent Psychiatry Nurse* 17.3 (2004): 93–103.

Joseph, Stephen, P. Alex Linley and George J. Harris. 'Understanding Positive Change Following Trauma and Adversity: Structural Clarification.' *Journal of Loss and Trauma* 10 (2005): 83–96.

Lazarus, Richard S. 'Coping Theory and Research: Past, Present, and Future.' *Psychosomatic Medicine* 55.3 (1993): 234–247.

Lebanon Higher Relief Council. 'Lebanon under Siege.' Page archived by TheWaybackMachine.org. Viewed 15 May 2016. http://archive.org/web/web.php.

Machel, Graca. 'For the Sake of Our Children.' *World Today* 57 (2001): 4–6.

Macksoud, Mona S. and Lawrence J. Aber. 'The War Experiences and Psychosocial Development of Children in Lebanon.' *Child Development* 67.1 (1996): 70–88.

Prince-Embury, Sandra. *Resiliency Scales for Adolescents: Profiles of Personal Strengths*. San Antonio, TX: Harcourt Assessments, 2006.

Punamaki, Raija-Leena, Katri Kanninen, Samir Qouta and Eyad El-Sarraj. 'The Role of Psychological Defences in Moderating between Trauma and Post-Traumatic Symptoms among Palestinian Men.' *International Journal of Psychology* 37.5 (2002): 286–296.

Qouta, Samir, Punamaki Raija-Leena, Thomas Miller and Eyad El-Sarraj. 'Does War Beget Child Aggression? Military Violence, Gender, Age and Aggressive Behavior in two Palestinian Samples.' *Aggressive Behavior* 34.3 (2008): 231–244.

Rasmusson, Elisabeth. 'Safeguarding the Children.' *Perspective: Humanitarian and International Affairs Magazine*, April 2011, 6–7.

Rogers, Mary J. and Grayson N. Holmbeck. 'Effects of Interparental Aggression on Children's Adjustment: The Moderating Role of Cognitive Appraisal and Coping.' *Journal of Family Psychology* 11.1 (1997): 125–130.

Rubin, Kenneth H., Patricia McDougall, Xinyin Chen, Anne Bowker and Joanne McKinnon. 'The Waterloo Longitudinal Project: Predicting Internalizing and Externalizing Problems in Adolescence.' *Development and Psychopathology* 7 (1995): 751–764.

Rubin, Kenneth H., William M. Bukowski and Jeffrey Parker. 'Peer Interactions, Relationships, and Groups.' *Handbook of Child Psychology: Vol. 3 Social, Emotional and Personality Development*, edited by William. E. Damon, 571–635. New York: Wiley, 1998.

Tayara, Rana. 'Resiliency and War Experiences: A Psychometric Study of the Lebanese Adolescent Experience of War.' *International Journal of Psychology and Behavioral Sciences* 3 (2013): 23–33.

United Nations High Commissioner for Refugees. Syria Regional Refugee Response [Internet]. UNHCR; 2014 *UNHCR.org*, 2014. Viewed 15 May 2016. http://data.unhcr.org/syrianrefugees/regional.php.

United Nations – General Assembly. 'Implementation of General Assembly Resolution 60/251 of 15 March 2006 Entitled "Human Rights Council": Opinions adopted by the Working Group on Arbitrary Detention.' 2 February 2007, *RefWorld.org*. Viewed 15 May 2016. http://www.refworld.org/docid/470b77b40.html.

Vygotsky, Lev S. *Mind in Society*. Cambridge, MA: Harvard University Press, 1978.

Yule, William, Derek Bolton, Orlee Udwin, Stephanie Boyle, Dominic O'Ryan and Julie Nurrish. 'The Long-Term Psychological Effects of a Disaster Experienced in Adolescence: I: The Incidence and Course of PTSD.' *Journal of Child Psychology and Psychiatry* 41.4 (2000): 503–505.

CHAPTER 5

The Resilient Journalist: Making Dollars and Sense

Lyn Barnes

Abstract

The role of journalism is to make sense of the world. Journalists tell stories to try to unravel the unbelievable, such as when planes mysteriously disappear, or a student decides to take a gun to his school and shoot his classmates. The journalist is the conjoint, informing people about what is known and what is not known. Today's graduate journalists must not only be competent in how to write a news story, take photographs, record video or an audio clip, but they must also be prepared to witness the most brutal scenes, sift out the most crucial information and show compassion – as well as meet never-ending deadlines. Then they must face the public, and often be abused for over-stepping the bounds of what is acceptable as they seek out news content. The symbiotic relationship between the press and the public is often tenuous. All too often journalists who cover tragedy and disaster are inexperienced at dealing with death and grief. Are they prepared adequately for being on the 'front lines' and the increasing stress that goes with the job? This chapter looks at using role-play as a way of teaching journalism students how to understand why people react differently to grief. Role-play has a two-fold function: to help graduates survive in an industry that progressively features violence and trauma content, and to learn how to protect themselves from distressing situations.

Keywords

journalism – reflective learning – role-play – trauma – trauma training

1 Trying to Make Meaning from Mayhem

Within days of Malaysia Airlines flight MH370 disappearing with 239 people on board, Danica Weeks had become a household name in Australasia. Her husband, Paul, was a passenger. Piers Morgan, 60 Minutes, and virtually every major news outlet around the world had interviewed the New Zealander, who now lives in Perth, Australia. Danica Weeks knew the media could help with

 | DOI:10.1163/9789004397576_007

her mission, to ensure her husband was not forgotten. As willing as she was to talk to the media, she soon became a news commodity, called on at every opportunity for comment. A young journalist contacted me because she was asked repeatedly by her editor to phone the young widow. She did not feel good about continually calling her but she dared not refuse. She began having nightmares, dreaming about the plane, swimming through victims' clothes, finding the wreckage in the sea. She wasn't the only one asking if all the stories about the missing plane were necessary. Was the media seeking to make meaning, to soothe the traumatised public of worry and fear in the wake and aftermath of the disappearance, or was it for the sake of yet another front-page story?

Whether it is the coverage of a murder, a natural disaster or a horrendous tragedy, journalism plays a fundamental role in helping us understand what is happening. Journalists construct meaning in the public domain through the complex process of representation, interpretation, and construction of reality. Often this involves journalism mediating reality then interacting with the public sphere across national boundaries.[1] Sometimes this is done by constantly retelling a story in different ways or adding a detail here or there, which helps the audience adjust to the shock, denial, and anger.

Now that we live in a culture of grief, as Carolyn Kitch asserts, journalism performs the rituals of grief and mourning for the public.[2] By personalising stories and focusing on a relative of a victim, journalists can make the most unbelievable stories more real – and the audience gets to experience pain at a safe arm's length. In today's society, the public has a need for heuristics: it wants explanations and possible causes. People want to know who was affected and how, yet are grateful they were not involved. Kitch sees the positive in such news stories, which she suggests, memorialise people.

Many journalists face ethical dilemmas when confronted with grief. As Kim Walsh-Childers, Norman Lewis, and Jeffrey Neely explain, journalists are expected to provide valuable information to help the public understand and respond appropriately to an unquestionably newsworthy and impactful event, while at the same time minimising harm to people who have suffered an almost unfathomable trauma.[3]

1 Verica Rupar, 'Journalism and Meaning-Making: Mapping the Field of Study,' *Journalism and Meaning-Making: Reading the Newspaper*, ed. Verica Rupar (Claskill, UK: Hampton Press, 2010), 1–12.

2 Carolyn Kitch, 'A News of Feeling as Well as Fact: Mourning and Memorial in American Newsmagazines,' *Journalism* 1 (2000): 171–195.

3 Kim Walsh-Childers, Norman P. Lewis and Jeffrey Neely, 'Listeners, not Leeches: What Virginia Tech Survivors Needed from Journalists,' *Journal of Mass Media Ethics* 26 (2011): 201.

Jordan Yentzer queries why we must 'incessantly repeat the news of a crisis,' which he refers to as 'parroting.' He argues that the 'parrot' represents a failure to adequately cope with a disaster, crisis, or rupture.

> Can we address traumatic events without naively repeating or parroting them? If not, how can we work more carefully in the face of crises so as to responsibly maintain an understanding of their severity?[4]

Yentzer refers in particular to the December 2012 Sandy Hook High Elementary School in Newtown, Connecticut, where 26 died in one of the deadliest mass shootings of pupils and teachers. School shootings are still incomprehensible to most people, so it is often up to journalists to try to make sense of a situation where there is no meaning, where the magnitude and meaninglessness are overwhelming.

As with the Virginia Tech rampage in 2007, when 32 students and faculty members were killed, hundreds of journalists were on the scene within hours. An event such as Sandy Hook encourages an influx of journalists from around the world and endless media calls to victims' families. The media want its audience to believe that it is making meaning but, just by being there en masse, representatives of the media can damage survivors. Walsh-Childers and colleagues suggest that even those journalists who adhere to ethical codes that urge professionals to treat victims with respect can unwittingly create harm simply through their sheer numbers.[5] That is because 'parroting' often requires returning to sources for more details and follow-up stories, as with Danica Weeks.

Therefore, simply gathering and reporting information may cause further harm and discomfort to victims. A reflective journalist will hopefully question his or her behaviour. Is she or he simply repeating information for sensational headlines, or is the journalist's role to soothe the concerns of readers?

2 Profit Motives and Public Hunger

For a story to be 'newsworthy' it must be immediate, dramatic and novel.[6] Traumatic events therefore provide the ideal media fodder and in turn revenue for

---

4 Jordan Yentzer, 'The Responsibility of the Parrot: Crisis, Response and Sandy Hook' (paper presented at the *Trauma Theory and Practice, 4th Global Conference*, Prague, Czech Republic, March 2014).

5 Walsh-Childers, Lewis and Neely, 'Listeners, not Leeches: What Virginia Tech Survivors Needed from Journalists,' 201.

6 Eileen Berrington and Ann Jemphrey, 'Pressure on the Press: Reflections on Reporting Tragedy,' *Journalism* 4 (2003): 228.

media moguls constantly struggling to make a profit in a time of change. It is convenient that bad news sells so well, as such cheap content is easy to source. The public also appears to have an enormous appetite for trauma-related stories. These stories are usually simplified and personalised, to encourage readers to identify with the characters or to make judgements about them.[7] Whether it is to make sense of situations or out of natural curiosity, there is a hunger for such coverage. Frank Ochberg describes the public as gluttonous for violent news and trauma coverage as unbalanced.[8] He envisages trauma news as three acts, all of which involve stories he believes must be told: Act One, he describes as the lurid and alluring traumatic event; Act Two, the hard but hopeful path from victim to survivor, and finally; Act Three, the struggle to find meaning when there is none, when something evil has occurred.[9]

Ochberg contends that we are programmed from childhood about good and evil with fairy tales, and that the move towards more violent images and the coverage of extreme events is implicit in human survival. Stories about victims, he suggests, could be considered as fairy tales for adults with heroes and villains. Ochberg says we need to hear them to help prepare ourselves for the unexpected and the subsequent sensations of shock and fear. 'We take in pictures of predators and predation, of monster and mayhem, so that we have templates in the brain when real danger strikes.'[10] Based on this reasoning, the psychiatrist-turned-trauma science specialist believes 'it is not inhuman and not depraved to have an appetite for violence,'[11] but it is simply part of our struggle for survival. We need mental representation of extreme events, he adds. For that reason, Ochberg understands why editors tend to follow the premise 'if it bleeds, it leads' and feature images of accidents and disasters.

> Competition for audience attention is part of media business, and we the audience attend to violence. We always have, always will, and *must*. Act One of any factual story about crime, cruelty, violence or trauma will create arousal, interest and paradoxical emotion. The only time a trauma story is pure horror is when it is about us.[12]

7 Ibid.
8 Frank M. Ochberg, 'Three Acts of Trauma News,' 1999, viewed 20 July, 2014, http://www.giftfromwithin.org/pdf/threeact.pdf.
9 Ibid.
10 Ibid.
11 Ibid.
12 Ibid.

To appeal to readers, it appears a news story must incorporate emotion because, as Ochberg admits, he, like other readers, has become jaded and needs more 'novelty, immediacy and consequence to be riveted by a trauma story.[13]

Trauma stories are often termed human-interest stories because of their shared universal news values. They are easy to read and understand and therefore have become ubiquitous. That is because journalists tend to focus on the last scene of Ochberg's Act One, the ritual of interviewing the grieving while the 'trauma is still hot,' to capture the 'compelling image of grief.'[14]

Ochberg would prefer that journalists waited until Act Two, once the initial shock has passed. Rather than focus on the 'victim' and all the negative connotations associated with the term, he believes the stories should be about the 'survivor' and recovery. In the early stages, after a traumatic event, he argues that victims are often in a fog, and are therefore unreliable witnesses. 'The physiology that helps us fight and flee also distorts perception.'[15] He would prefer survivor stories lead the news and disaster stories be expanded to include reflections by survivors. Ochberg believes Act Two stories are just as compelling and newsworthy as Act One's alluring pieces, but are harder to find and more difficult to format. Instead, Act One stories are often overdone and sensationalised. He believes we have become addicted to Act One and dismissive of Act Two as 'saccharine or simply not newsworthy.'[16]

There is more support for this argument. Research suggests that readers prefer the more traditional or 'episodic' framed stories about isolated incidents, as opposed to 'thematic' framing, in which stories focus on the bigger picture.[17] Also, the public's appetite for sensationalism creates a market for products gained from insensitive and intrusive tactics that some journalists employ.[18] So it appears that as long as sensation and intrusion-based stories continue to sell newspapers, journalists will remain under pressure to produce material to meet demand.[19] Sometimes the stress on journalists is exacerbated by the need to beat the competition and keep their employers happy. Folker Hanusch

13 Ibid.
14 Ochberg, 'Three Acts of Trauma News.'
15 Ibid.
16 Ibid.
17 Sara Tiegreen and Elana Newman, 'How News is Framed,' *Fact Sheet*, Dart Center for Journalism & Trauma, University of Columbia, New York, viewed 26 July 2014, http://dartcenter.org/content/how-news-is-framed#.U9dNu4CSwo8.
18 Linda Kay, Rosemary Reilly, Elyse Amend and Terry Kyle, 'Between a Rock and a Hard Place,' *Journalism Studies* 12 (2011): 440–455.
19 Berrington and Jemphrey, 'Pressure on the Press: Reflections on Reporting Tragedy,' 239.

attributes this to the fact that news organisations are competing now more than ever before for the attention of audiences.[20] Eileen Berrington and Ann Jemphrey would agree:

> Twin pressures impact on journalists reporting deaths – the personal and the commercial. They have the worry of banging on doors and intruding, compounded by the pressure of meeting deadlines.[21]

Ochberg would argue that it is also because we, the audience, have short attention spans that we overdose on Act One stories. Act Two stories are often relegated to the feature section or to a magazine and the message lost because the message of hope, patience, and resilience are not as gripping. Act Three stories, he proposes, are also often overlooked; those are stories where there is no chance of healing. Examples he cites are the Holocaust, the Rwandan massacres, and the annihilation of a family by a depraved psychopath. Ochberg would no doubt have included the subsequent mass school murders that have happened since he wrote his seminal essay. Even though these stories make no sense and nothing good comes of them, he believes they must be told. But these stories Ochberg insists must be told simply, with just the facts, as he believes 'every piece of human history has a purpose and lesson.'[22] He attributes blame for the imbalance not only to the audience but also to media owners.

> When we, the audience, tire of the formulaic, repetitive treatment of trauma in the news, the formula will change. But we may not tire. We may be destined by biology to feed endlessly on other peoples' horror, distorting our perception and understanding of reality. And if that, indeed, is true, a new journalism and new journalist is needed to help us overcome ourselves.[23]

3 Dealing with the Pressure

Journalism students may benefit from experiencing people in various stages of grief and realise there is a number of steps to recovery. While victims are still in

20 Folker Hanusch, 'Graphic Death in the New Media: Present or Absent?' *Mortality* 13 (2008): 301–317.

21 Berrington and Jemphrey, 'Pressure on the Press: Reflections on Reporting Tragedy,' 239.

22 Ochberg, 'Three Acts of Trauma News.'

23 Ibid.

a state of shock or disbelief, which is often followed by emotional release, they provide the most colourful content. It is immediately after a death or disaster that journalists are most often sent out, or asked to phone relatives, 'to get them while they're hot.'[24] But this is also a time when an intrusion can do the most damage, sometimes interrupting the grieving process.[25] Walsh-Childers and her fellow researchers assert that journalists should be taught to distinguish between those people who are emotionally ready to tell their stories and those who should be left alone for a few hours.[26]

So it could be that journalists well prepared to deal with trauma may play a vital role in changing the culture of newsrooms. A reflective journalist who understands grief is more likely to question what they are asked to do and know how to approach a trauma situation from a different perspective. He or she will realise that victims should not be used as a means to an end, nor bullied and pushed. Not only is it unethical but, as Walsh-Childers and colleagues found, the outcome is seldom positive … 'those [journalists] whose behaviour created a sense of sincere rapport won the interviews and cooperation they needed to get their stories, both immediately and in the months that followed.'[27]

4 Confusion with Codes of Ethics

As part of journalism training, all journalists are taught to adhere to their profession's code of ethics. One global message is to minimise harm. But as Ian Richards highlights, most codes are riddled with inconsistencies and are open to different interpretations, for example, what does 'minimize harm' really mean, he asks?[28] As illustrated here, simply having a media circus at the scene of a mass murder can further traumatise people. Most journalism codes of ethics also refer to 'respecting private grief and personal privacy.' But Richards queries what the words 'respect' and 'privacy' actually mean? In New Zealand and Australia, the code includes the statement: 'Journalists

24 Ian Richards, 'Encountering Death for the First Time,' *Australian Journalism Review* 16 (1994): 119.

25 Jolyon Sykes and Kerry Green, 'The Danger of Dealing with Journalists' (paper presented at the Australia and New Zealand Communications Association Conference, Brisbane, July 2003).

26 Walsh-Childers, Lewis and Neely, 'Listeners, not Leeches: What Virginia Tech Survivors Needed from Journalists.'

27 Ibid., 202.

28 Richards, 'Ethics: Journalists and Victims,' 155.

have the right to resist compulsion to intrude.' But, as Richards points out, how does the individual journalist exercise the 'right to resist compulsion' when a chief reporter is insisting that the journalist not give up on getting an interview from a grieving relative? There is an enormous push-pull effect on some journalists who are reluctant to return to the office without a story and ideally a photograph, or they will be made to feel they failed. Some have openly been told they are not doing their job if they do not find a contact and get some direct quotes.

5 Crossing the Line

Although ethics training is now routine in most journalism schools worldwide, it is often theoretical. It is not until the graduate is out in the field, usually alone, that he or she may have to grapple with such situations. Richards cautions that it is when they are operating under the pressures of reporting stories involving trauma that most journalists may, at most, only glance at a code of ethics.

> The reality is that most journalists respond in ways which enable them to meet the demands and expectations of those of greater seniority in their organisation – which mean, ultimately, those who employ them.[29]

He continues ...

> even if they are committed to behaving ethically, the best-equipped graduates may still encounter difficulty in applying principles taught in the classroom to the various ethical dilemmas of working journalism.[30]

A more practical approach to ethics and trauma reporting may encourage journalists on the job to think carefully about the repercussions. It may also empower them to speak up if they feel uncomfortable or resist pressure, which is likely to continue with the increasing demand for trauma-related stories.

> As ratings and circulation follow the content of the story rather than the manner in which it is prepared, there has been considerable pressure on

29 Ibid., 156.
30 Ibid., 156.

> individual journalists "to bend the rules" to get the story with the most audience impact.[31]

Even experienced journalists feel the pressure at times, especially if they are out of touch with reporting from the scene of an incident. Veteran BBC reporter Colin Brazier crossed the line at the site of the downed Malaysian airline flight MH17 when he rifled through personal belongings of victims. As he was doing his piece to camera he admitted, 'We shouldn't be doing this really,' but continued to handle a young girl's belongings, wallet, and keys. Following criticism, Brazier said he was caught in the moment and because other journalists were rummaging through baggage he 'foolishly took that as precedent.'[32] He also blamed the fact that he had been desk bound for some time. Sometimes even the wording or descriptions journalists use at times can cross the line. With any news story, there should always be a point to using description or detail. It is questionable whether this extract from the *New York Times* has any news value other than to sensationalise, especially when children are involved.

> Bodies lying in the field struck strange, unnatural shapes in the tall grasses, many naked but for their shoes. Some were nestled together among piles of open suitcases, including a man in a mint-colored T-shirt lying near a woman in torn jeans whose right arm was thrown up over her head as if she were trying to protect herself. Others lay alone, like the tiny girl, probably no older than 3, dressed in a red T-shirt without pants.[33]

Certainly, description and detail are sometimes necessary, especially in Ochberg's Act Three stories of evil, for example, regarding the Holocaust or after the atomic bomb was dropped on Hiroshima. Had it not been for John Hersey's personalising and poignant portrayal in *The New Yorker*,[34] Americans may never have realised the consequences of a nuclear weapon that killed more than 140,000 Japanese and maimed hundreds more.

---

31 Ibid., 150.

32 Michael Koziol, 'Sky News Journalist Colin Brazier Apologises for Rummaging through Belongings of MH17 Victims,' *Sydney Morning Herald*, 23 July 2014, viewed 27 July 2014, http://www.smh.com.au/world/sky-news-journalist-colin-brazier-apologises-for-rummaging-through-belongings-of-mh17-victims-20140723-zvwwx.html.

33 Peter Baker, 'With Jet Strike, War in Ukraine Is Felt Globally,' *New York Times*, 19 July 2014, viewed 27 July 2014, http://www.nytimes.com/2014/07/20/world/europe/with-jets-fall-war-in-ukraine-is-felt-globally.html?_r=0.

34 John Hersey, 'Hiroshima,' *The New Yorker*, August 31, 1946, viewed 12 July 2014, http://www.newyorker.com/magazine/1946/08/31/hiroshima.

6 Bringing Death to Life

Not all stories about anguish and disaster do damage, as Hersey proved. Having their stories told sensitively and accurately can help survivors reconnect with their lives and community and validate their feelings about the event.[35]

So how do we ensure that graduate journalists have the skills to deal with victims and their families in a manner that is positive for all involved? A study by Elyse Amend, Linda Kay, and Rosemary Reilly drew on the links between the ethical dilemmas journalists face when covering trauma and violence and explored how a journalist's actions are tied to his or her level of training and preparedness.[36] Debate continues about the best way to learn trauma skills. Some would argue that such skills cannot be taught, but that they can only be experienced, and with experience comes competency and resiliency. Others totally disagree; is it ethical to practise on the public?

The Dart Centre for Journalism and Trauma, based at Columbia University in New York, has become a resource base for trauma journalism. As Bruce Shapiro, the centre director points out, a business reporter is seldom sent out to do a story without some background knowledge, so a young reporter covering a death should be equipped with some basic trauma skills. Death affects everyone and trauma is part of life, he adds. Shapiro, along with Ari Goldman, a professor of journalism at Columbia University, believes students must be properly prepared to deal with death and dying. As representatives of Dart, they suggest that the best way to do this is to make death come alive. They recommend that all journalism students gain experience in talking to the bereaved, and that they need to know how to cover a murder or suicide correctly.

Goldman suggests a good place to start is by having students write obituaries, then moving beyond that to discussing the diversity of death rituals, for example, the concept of open caskets or embalming.[37] He advocates sending students in pairs to funerals of people outside their tradition or culture, or visiting a morgue. A further step is to write about memorials related to death without becoming too close to those affected, for example, a statue or cross on the side of the road. The next step is to interview someone associated with death, for

---

35 Sallyanne Duncan and Jackie Newton, 'How Do You Feel? Preparing Novice Reporters for the Death Knock,' *Journalism Practice* 4 (2010): 439–453.

36 Elyse Amend, Linda Kay and Rosemary C. Reilly, 'Journalism on the Spot: Ethical Dilemmas When Covering Trauma and the Implications for Journalism Education,' *Journal of Mass Media Ethics* 27 (2012): 236.

37 Ari Goldman, 'Covering Death and Dying,' Lecture at Dart Centre for Journalism and Trauma, Columbia Journalism School, New York, June 29, 2012.

example, interviewing a student whose mother is terminally ill – and teaching the students to always be prepared for the unexpected. This way, suggests Goldman, students find out how to talk to grieving people, and how they might respond if someone they are interviewing bursts into tears for example. Slowly but surely, journalism students learn to manage their emotions and identify their vulnerabilities.

An important aspect of dealing with grief and trauma is being aware that it can take its toll and build in intensity over time. Therefore, self-care is encouraged to recognise stress. Taking the time to process trauma is encouraged as it can prevent cumulative stress, mistakes in reporting as well as maintain a creativity that is needed to produce good, accurate stories.[38]

7 The Role of Role-Play

The pressure on journalists is not likely to ease up in the foreseeable future and the increase in social media will not help. The profession faces even more pressure with the widespread use of mobile devices that make the newsgathering process instantaneous.[39] For this reason, Linda Kay, Rosemary Reilly, Elyse Amend, and Terry Kyle advocate the role of professional reflective practice for both the public good and the professionalism of journalism. Role-play complements traditional lectures, not only by reinforcing learning, but also by catering to the different ways people learn.[40] It involves having people act out particular roles, creating incidents or hypothetical situations through actions and mannerisms in a risk-free situation. Role-play is an example of experiential learning, as it is activity related and learner-centred. It provides an opportunity for students to examine and explore their responses. Students participate as well as observe their peers, thereby learning from the experience. Afterwards, learning is reinforced through sharing their responses and reactions. Amend and her colleagues found that information is imprinted in a powerful way through the use of simulations in the classroom.[41]

Role-play is an established model of teaching and learning that has been introduced to a range of disciplines including education, medicine and nursing

38 Patrice Keats and Marla Buchanan, 'Addressing the Effects of Assignment Stress Injury,' *Journalism Practice* 3 (2009): 165.

39 Kay, Reilly, Amend and Kyle, 'Between a Rock and a Hard Place,' 453.

40 Kristine M. DeNeve and Mary J. Heppner, 'Role-Play Simulations: The Assessment of an Active Learning Technique and Comparisons with Traditional Lectures,' *Innovative Higher Education* 21 (1997): 231–246.

41 Amend, Kay and Reilly, 'Journalism on the Spot,' 246.

training, law, and social work. Researchers suggest that one of the reasons trauma training is not taught routinely is the lack of evidence about which model of teaching is most effective.[42] Other researchers disagree. Barry Richards and Gavin Rees point towards role-play as the most effective, low-cost way of achieving higher order learning and retaining valuable information.[43] Diane Billings advocates role-play in medical training because it addresses higher learning abilities, such as interpersonal skills, which do not come naturally. Role-play gives students the opportunity to refine their communication skills, identify feelings, develop problem-solving skills, collaborate, and make decisions.[44]

> Based on the principles of experiential learning, simulations of traumatic events can not only permit students to apply their theoretical knowledge but also develop the necessary interaction skills that characterise sensitive trauma reporting. They reveal the subtleties of empathetic human social interaction and are effective in building communication skills.[45]

It is well established that a range of problems can arise when ill-equipped journalists are faced with covering a traumatic event, from basic inaccuracies to serious ethical violations.[46] For young journalists, therefore, it is wise to practise in a safe space, because interviewing a grieving person involves many skills all at once. These skills include, for example: asking sensitive, appropriate questions; sometimes recording and taking notes at the same time; coping with time pressure and a deadline; identifying their own feelings and dealing with them; self-assessment (keeping their own emotions in check but also being aware when they are uncomfortable); assessing any risks (considering the situation they are in); realising the importance of double-checking facts; problem solving; making decisions; and sometimes, working as a team by collaborating with other journalists.

The Auckland University of Technology's journalism department employs professional actors to carry out role-plays with students. The scenarios are real-life experiences of former students who encountered similar traumatic

42 Sallyanne Duncan, 'Sadly Missed: The Death Knock News Story as a Personal Narrative of Grief,' *Journalism* 13 (2012): 439–453.

43 Barry Richards and Gavin Rees, 'The Management of Emotion in British Journalism,' *Media, Culture and Society* 33 (2011): 851–867.

44 Diana Billings, 'Role-Play Revisited,' *The Journal of Continuing Education in Nursing* 43 (2012): 201–202.

45 Amend, Kay and Reilly, 'Journalism on the Spot,' 247.

46 Walsh-Childers, Lewis and Neely, 'Listeners, not Leeches: What Virginia Tech Survivors Needed from Journalists.'

situations in their first year on the job. These include interviewing a grandfather whose grandson has drowned in his pool while in his care, a young woman who has witnessed a car accident and is extremely distressed, and an older woman who has been attacked by an intruder in her home. Each scenario has a 'back story,' which the students are to uncover during the 'interviews.' As with all news stories, they need to filter the information they are given, for example, the racist rant of the older woman. There are many distractions, especially if the students are not expecting responses such as tears or anger.

It is common to observe that students do not concentrate or listen carefully, a critical skill needed at any time with their work, but particularly when interviewing someone who is traumatised. Some students adhere to their set questions instead of responding to what victims say and can miss important points. Some lack basic empathic skills or are embarrassed and self-conscious about what to say, so avoid eye contact with interviewees and spend too much time looking down or writing notes. This often creates awkward silences and gaps in the conversation. An interesting observation, which the students identified themselves, was the surprise at their own reactions. Some felt emotional and did not know how to deal with that response. Another smiled, an inappropriate yet involuntary reaction, which he realised he would need to address before doing a 'real' trauma interview.

Role-play is also proving to be an excellent way of practising, perfecting, and endorsing the importance of not forgetting the basics, such as clearly identifying themselves and who they work for when they first meet people, an ethical must. Through making mistakes during role-plays the students also learn to check names and other vital details, which can cause further stress to victims if inaccurate.

Anxiety is often palpable during the role-plays, even though the students know they are 'interviewing' actors. Some researchers argue that anxiety is a key to reflective learning.[47] David Boud believes that reflection thrives on doubt and is hard won because it is 'associated with questioning, uncertainties, discrepancies and dissatisfactions.'[48] At the same time it is important that there is a balance with the experience, so the students are not anxious either. Some remarked afterwards that they never thought journalists would have to cover trauma, and it was not what they intended to do workwise. So

---

47 John Steel, Bill Carmichael, David Holmes, Marie Kinse, and Karen Sanders, 'Experiential Learning and Journalism Education: Lessons Learned in the Practice of Teaching Journalist,' *Education + Training* 49 (2007): 325–334.

48 David Boud, 'Avoiding the Traps: Seeking Good Practice in the Use of Self-Assessment and Reflection in Professional Courses,' *Social Work Education* 18 (1999): 123.

the exercises are also a reality check for some students who have an idealised impression of the profession.

The role-play programme at Auckland University of Technology has operated for three years and with only a modest budget to pay actors, there are sometimes five students in each 'interview.' Ideally it would be one-on-one and no more than three. What is observable in bigger groups is that weak students who lack confidence can 'disappear' easily and not participate. The opposite can also happen. In an earlier study by Boud, along with David Walker, the pair found that the dynamics of a group could take over, which can then influence attitudes and behaviour negatively. 'People are drawn into it, and often act in a way that is contrary to what they might do alone.'[49] However, in reality, as with real-life scenarios discussed earlier in this chapter, there may be a number of journalists on the scene, for example, vying for the story, so they cannot afford to 'disappear.' Competition for the first story or photograph, along with pressure from editors to meet deadlines, increases pressure on journalists 'to get the story.' Having several students in a group, all after the same story, creates a teachable moment about the implications of 'pack mentality' and how it can arise, as happened with the Colin Brazier incident regarding Flight MH17.

More fine-tuning is needed with the role-plays, for example, whether to film the students so they can watch themselves later in private and identify their strengths and weaknesses. In the past, we have had students from digital media courses film the students. Next year we may have students film each other with smart phones, to avoid being distracted by a 'real' camera. Several students commented during the debriefings that they felt self-conscious with the camera in the room and that it made them more inclined to make mistakes. Other observational methods could be less intrusive. It is interesting to observe physical responses, for example, whether the students' body language and responses are appropriate, or alternatively, if they involuntarily employ avoidance behaviours, such as bowing their heads and resisting eye contact.

Another issue for further discussion is the role of the teacher in role-plays and how much should he or she be involved both during and after the 'interviews.' David Schön suggests teachers should act only as coaches, rather than as teachers. He recommends interrupting a session if a student makes a mistake, and the actor goes into 'freeze' mode.[50] That is understandable with medical

49 David Boud and David Walker, 'Promoting Reflection in Professional Courses: the Challenge of Context,' *Studies in Higher Education* 23 (1998): 198.

50 Donald Schön, *The Reflective Practitioner* (US: Basic Books, 1983).

students, where life and death situations might be involved, but it would interrupt the flow of an interview. So far, we have not done this mainly because of the limited time available for trauma training.[51] Instead, we ask the actors to step out of their roles at the end of the 'interviews' to give immediate feedback to students. This has proved extremely worthwhile, as the actors, who regularly work with the local medical school, are experienced in giving positive and negative feedback. This initiative, a suggestion of one of the actors, also relieves any tension the students may feel if they encounter anger or other emotions. Teachers can also give feedback and make suggestions at this time, but are asked to be encouraging.

8 The Debriefing

The Dart Centre for Journalism and Trauma makes it clear that preparation, implementation, and debriefing are crucial elements in any role-play. Students at Auckland University of Technology are asked to fill in a questionnaire with a range of open and closed questions as the starting point to the debriefing. This is followed by a general discussion. However, this segment of the training needs to be developed more. General verbal feedback is always surprisingly good but the students seldom go beyond saying that it was a good opportunity to analyse their interviewing techniques. Boud believes that leaving time to reflect is not enough,[52] but it is encouraging to know that reflection can obviously occur when circumstances are less than ideal.[53]

9 Conclusion

The best feedback about using role-play as a way of teaching trauma literacy comes once the graduates have been working for a few months. Such feedback is usually in the form of an email of thanks, grateful that they had some basic skills to do their first trauma interview and managed it well. There are still many areas to refine, for example, group size, whether to film the students or not, use of props, teacher involvement and ensuring positive self-learning through an effective debriefing session. But overall, this form of experiential learning appears to be positive for everyone involved. Developing practical evaluation and assessment

---

51 Ibid.

52 Boud, 'Avoiding the Traps,' 125.

53 Boud and Walker, 'Promoting Reflection,' 205.

measures are now required to confirm the initial outcomes of role-play as an effective method of quality reflection.

True success will come when enough graduates feel strong enough to say no if they do not agree with what they are being asked to do without feeling that their jobs may be in jeopardy, and when they feel comfortable about asking for help if they are feeling stressed by their work. That change may come when they ask themselves whether they are simply being 'parrots' and hassling a victim for yet another interview for a story, or whether they are making meaning for an audience that needs further explanation of something that is unfathomable without their help. At present, as Ochberg suggests, trauma news is skewed and distorted, but this is not only the responsibility of journalists but editors, media owners and ultimately, the audience.[54] Until there is some change, Richards warns that the onus for ethical behaviour continues to be placed on the individual journalist.[55]

Bibliography

Amend, Elyse, Linda Kay and Rosemary C. Reilly. 'Journalism on the Spot: Ethical Dilemmas when Covering Trauma and the Implications for Journalism Education.' *Journal of Mass Media Ethics* 27 (2012): 235–247.

Baker, Peter. 'With Jet Strike, War in Ukraine is Felt Globally,' *New York Times*, 19 July, 2014. Viewed 27 July 2014. http://www.nytimes.com/2014/07/20/world/europe/with-jets-fall-war-in-ukraine-is-felt-globally.html?_r=0.

Berrington, Eileen and Ann Jemphrey. 'Pressure on the Press: Reflections on Reporting Tragedy.' *Journalism* 4 (2003): 225–248.

Billings, Diana. 'Role-Play Revisited.' *The Journal of Continuing Education in Nursing* 43 (2012): 201–202.

Boud, David. 'Avoiding the Traps: Seeking Good Practice in the Use of Self-Assessment and Reflection in Professional Courses.' *Social Work Education* 18 (1999): 121–132.

Boud, David and David Walker. 'Promoting Reflection in Professional Courses: The Challenge of Context.' *Studies in Higher Education* 23 (1998): 191–206.

DeNeve, Kristine M. and Mary J. Heppner. 'Role-Play Simulations: The Assessment of an Active Learning Technique and Comparisons with Traditional Lectures.' *Innovative Higher Education* 21 (1997): 231–246.

54 Ochberg, 'Three Acts of Trauma News,' 1999.

55 Richards, 'Ethics: Journalists and Victims,' 151.

Duncan, Sallyanne. 'Sadly Missed: The Death Knock News Story as a Personal Narrative of Grief.' *Journalism* 13 (2012): 589–603.

Duncan, Sallyanne and Jackie Newton. 'How Do You Feel? Preparing Novice Reporters for the Death Knock.' *Journalism Practice* 4 (2010): 439–453.

Goldman, Ari. 'Covering Death and Dying.' Lecture at Dart Centre for Journalism and Trauma, Columbia Journalism School, New York, June 29, 2012.

Hanusch, Folker. 'Graphic Death in the New Media: Present or Absent?' *Mortality* 13 (2008): 301–317.

Hersey, John. 'Hiroshima,' *The New Yorker*, August 31, 1946. Viewed 12 July 2014. http://www.newyorker.com/magazine/1946/08/31/hiroshima.

Kay, Linda, Rosemary Reilly, Elyse Amend and Terry Kyle. 'Between a Rock and a Hard Place.' *Journalism Studies* 12 (2011): 440–455.

Keats, Patrice and Marla Buchanan. 'Addressing the Effects of Assignment Stress Injury.' *Journalism Practice* 3 (2009): 162–177.

Kitch, Carolyn. 'A News of Feeling as well as Fact: Mourning and Memorial in American Newsmagazines.' *Journalism* 1 (2000): 171–195.

Koziol, Michael. 'Sky News Journalist Colin Brazier Apologises for Rummaging through Belongings of MH17 Victims,' *Sydney Morning Herald*, 23 July 2014. Viewed 27 July 2014.http://www.smh.com.au/world/sky-news-journalist-colin-brazier-apologises-for-rummaging-through-belongings-of-mh17-victims-20140723-zvwwx.html.

Ochberg, Frank M. 'Three Acts of Trauma News.' 1999. Viewed 20 July 2014. http://www.giftfromwithin.org/pdf/threeact.pdf.

Richards, Barry and Gavin Rees. 'The Management of Emotion in British Journalism.' *Media, Culture & Society* 33 (2011): 851–867.

Richards, Ian. 'Ethics: Journalists and Victims.' *Journalism: Theory and Practice*, edited by Myles Breen, 141–161. Sydney: Macleay Press, 1998.

Richards, Ian. 'Encountering Death for the First Time.' *Australian Journalism Review* 16 (1994): 115–120.

Rupar, Verica. 'Journalism and Meaning-Making: Mapping the Field of Study.' *Journalism and Meaning-Making: Reading the Newspaper*, edited by Verica Rupar, 1–12. Claskill, UK: Hampton Press, 2010.

Sanders, Karen. 'Experiential Learning and Journalism Education: Lessons Learned in the Practice of Teaching Journalism.' *Education + Training* 49 (2007): 325–334.

Schön, Donald. *The Reflective Practitioner*. New York: Basic Books, 1983.

Steel, John, Bill Carmichael, David Holmes, Marie Kinse and Karen Sanders. 'Experiential Learning and Journalism Education: Lessons Learned in the Practice of Teaching Journalist.' *Education + Training* 49 (2007): 325–334.

Sykes, Jolyon and Kerry Green. 'The Danger of Dealing with Journalists.' Paper presented at the Australia and New Zealand Communications Association Conference, Brisbane, July 2003.

Tiegreen, Sara and Elana Newman. 'How News is Framed.' *Dart Center for Journalism and Trauma.* Viewed 26 July 2014. http://dartcenter.org/content/how-news-is-framed#.U9dNu4CSwo8.

Walsh-Childers, Kim, Norman P. Lewis and Jeffrey Neely. 'Listeners, not Leeches: What Virginia Tech Survivors Needed from Journalists.' *Journal of Mass Media Ethics* 26 (2011): 191–205.

Yentzer, Jordan. 'The Responsibility of the Parrot: Crisis, Response and Sandy Hook.' Paper presented at the *Trauma Theory and Practice, 4th Global Conference*, Prague, Czech Republic, March 2014.

CHAPTER 6

The Public Dimension of Privatized Trauma: Impact and Response

Joan Simalchik

Abstract

In its 1984 report, *Torture in the Eighties*, Amnesty International called torture 'the twentieth century epidemic.' Widely practiced and institutionally sanctioned, torture and state repression created *circles of silence* enshrouding individuals, families and communities. Officially denied, torture became an open secret creating conditions of cognitive dissonance for both victimized individuals and the wider society. Many refugees fleeing these regimes found asylum in countries of the Global North where trauma treatment centres were developed. Later, emerging from state dictatorships, new governments in periods of democratic reclamation negotiated the memory of past atrocities according to their own particular political exigencies. Incorporating Ignacio Martin Baro's theory of psychosocial destruction and Paulo Freire's notion of critical consciousness, this chapter will discuss the relationship between legacies of trauma and how individual and collective traumatic memory has been managed in countries after dictatorship, i.e. Chile and Brazil and in countries of exile, i.e. Canada.

Keywords

public and political trauma – torture – traumatic displacement

1 Introduction

Many countries in Latin America, such as Chile and Brazil, have been engaged in long periods of democratic transitions following conditions of dictatorship and war. Frequently, these transition governments have been the result of pacted agreements between divided constituencies in newly emergent, but unreconciled, civil societies. Prolonged exposure to repression, organized violence and war produced cultures of fear and present psychosocial obstacles to the establishment of good governance and a human rights culture.

 | DOI:10.1163/9789004397576_008

These transitions from cultures of fear provoke inquiry on behalf of those who survived them. How do those who had been victimized experience this psychosocial impact? How does this affect the work undertaken with torture survivors in both their homelands and in countries of asylum?

Additionally, questions remain about how the past influences the present society and culture. How does the legacy of state violence affect transitions? How does the process of democratization frame power relations within a context of contested memory and meaning? What is the nature of the problem of historical and current violence in the Americas, especially in Chile and Brazil? How do these particular contexts influence traumatic recovery?

2 The Legacy

In 1976, Canadian churches organized a fact-finding mission to Latin America that was conducted by three federal Ministers of Parliament from the Progressive Conservative, Liberal, and New Democratic political parties. They titled their report *One Gigantic Prison* in a trenchant comment on the state of the region. They found widespread institutionalized repressive measures utilized by national security states that included torture, disappearance, execution, imprisonment, forced exile, and internal relegation. These tactics were generally utilized, alone or in combination, as part of a continuum of repression that suppressed basic democratic rights. The mission provided a series of recommendations that included urging recognition of the atrocities by the United Nations and its member states and an opening of borders to accept refugees from these dictatorships.

Persecution was expressly designed to assist regimes that could not be freely elected to govern through force and these practices affected individuals, families, communities and society as a whole. The objectives were clearly intended to pacify and subjugate entire populations and to eliminate active and potential dissidents by creating radical disruptions of civil society. Systems of organized state violence were designed to attack the body politic, but the entry wound would be made through the individual subject.

Torture, in particular, was devised as a calculated, planned and systematic operation carried out by state functionaries. Words fail to convey the horrors that were, and continue to be, devised. Torture is brutality inflicted with the purpose of subduing potential or real opponents and incapacitating resistance. The purpose was not to execute the body but the mind, spirit and soul. Often medical intervention by physicians kept victims alive through the ordeal, although many did die under conditions of extreme duress. The practice was designed to inflict severe physical and psychological harm and then release the victim back to the community as an embodied warning to others.

Officially practiced but also officially denied, these human rights crimes produced cultures of fear. Norbert Lechner in 'Some People Die of Fear: Fear as a Political Problem' ascribes the origin of the term *culture of fear* to political scientist Guillermo O'Donnell. It refers to 'the wholesale, every day experience of human rights abuse. We experience the imprint of authoritarianism as a culture of fear.'[1]

Ignacio Martin-Baro, a Jesuit psychologist working in El Salvador, explored the meaning of state terror and its effect on people and culture.[2] He developed a method for understanding and resisting what he termed *psychosocial destruction* leading to trauma. Three fundamental elements inform the notion of *psychosocial trauma*: organized violence; institutionalized lies, and social polarization.

These three elements weave a complex web of denial among individuals, their families, and the communities in which they live creating what Martin-Baro named *circles of silence*. Under conditions of war and dictatorship, these serve to obscure daily reality and ensure that society does not have a reflective mirror in which to authenticate its experience.[3] Cognitive dissonance occurs when people are said to disappear, when massacres are unreported, and official stories evade or obfuscate the truth. There is little, if any, social space to express what is known to take place. These elements work on multiple and impermanent levels, implicating individuals and through their social actions, communities.

Vamik Volkan, a Turkish psychiatrist working in the United States, raises important issues regarding the psychopolitical journeys of trauma and how massive acts of cruelty such as torture lead to shared shame, fears, and difficulties in mourning. The removal of oppressive regimes or the breakup of political systems creates transgenerational trauma with 'malignant and destructive consequences.'[4] Without an institutional response and acknowledgement of

---

1 Norbert Lechner, *Fear at the Edge: State, Terror and Resistance in Latin America*, eds. Juan Corradi, Patricia Weiss Fagen, Manuel Antonia Garreton (Berkeley: University of Berkeley Press, 1992), 26.

2 Ignacio Martin-Baro was one of the five Jesuits who, along with their housekeeper and her daughter, were murdered by the Salvadoran army in November 1989 on the campus of the University of Central America.

3 Ignacio Martin-Baro, *Writings for a Liberation Psychology* (Cambridge, Ma: Harvard University Press, 1994).

4 Vamik Volkan, 'Large-Group Narcissism and Political Leaders,' *A Special Issue of Psychiatric Annals* 39 (2009) viewed 23 May 2015, http://www.vamikvolkan.com/Large-group-Narcissism-and-Political-Leaders.php.

the public dimension of human rights crimes, the impact remains privatized, individualized, and injurious.

3 Resistance

Despite the massive assault on civil society, resistance efforts were undertaken that challenged the repression and incrementally expanded the social space available for democracy. People organized and acted; they challenged circles of silence, overcoming fear and shame. Associations of relatives of the disappeared were initiated in Chile, Brazil, Argentina, and many other Latin American countries that demanded regimes disclose what happened to their family members. Survivors of torture and massacres provided testimonial evidence of human rights atrocities that was then relayed to the United Nations and international human rights organizations. People claimed democratic and human rights that had been violently abrogated and they demanded justice.

The resistance took many forms including protests, strikes, and, in a few countries, militant, armed, organized opposition. Incipient civil society organizations laid claim to their social roles. The mystique around cultures of fear was punctured enough to bring to a close systems of dictatorship and war. But in these pacted negotiated transitions, the ensuing structural formations and/or the political agency of the transition leadership proved to be too weak or incapable of fully facing the past and addressing consequent justice issues.

By the 1990s, many countries, Argentina, Chile, Uruguay, El Salvador, and Guatemala to name a few, each in its own way, began to emerge from dictatorship and/or open warfare and were subsequently defined as making the transition to democracy. Some states were declared to be democratic and others seemed to be mired in permanent states of transition.

4 Reparation and Renewal

Torture is widely practiced throughout the world. Recent studies have indicated that 50% of all countries, including 79% of the G-20 countries, continue to practice systematic torture despite a universal ban.[5] Sadly, in spite of United Nations Conventions and Amnesty International's campaigns, torture is still carried out in specific contexts in countries today, even by democratically

5 A. J. Carinci, et al., 'Chronic Pain in Torture Victims,' *Current Pain and Headache Reports* 14.2 (2010): 73–79.

elected governments. 'We tortured some folks,' President Barack Obama admitted in anticipation of the August 2014 U.S. Senate Report of CIA actions following 9/11.[6] For survivors, this fact destabilizes possibilities for safe and secure environments in which to process their past.

Perceptions of horror vary depending on contextual elements. For example, institutionalized torture that comes from within one's own country can be experienced very differently from isolated acts of torture perpetrated by non-state criminals. Slovo refers to work done with the South African Truth and Reconciliation project through which participants realized that apartheid was over and it was now time to face the losses endured, 'opening the floodgates of memory, most of which was full of the horrors of what they had witnessed.'[7]

The process of *de-privatizing* traumatic experiences becomes paramount for healing when individuals who were victimized continue to be made to bear their pain silently. Under conditions of war and dictatorship, threats to family and friends by perpetrators, fears of bystanders to corroborate atrocities, the seeming impossibility of proclaiming truth, all collude to maintain circles of silence. In post-dictatorship contexts the process of how projects move the private into a more public dimension determines whether the past will be contained and regulated or become unending intrusion.

De-privatizing implies the understanding of opposing meanings and rationalities that are legalized and normalized by people in power. The sanctioning of human rights crimes by the state in the past will have complex impact in the present and future of its citizens. As Agger and Jensen inquired in their study of dictatorship in Chile, '[H]ow much truth is necessary and how much can the public take?'[8] When truth has been obscured or deliberately denied, when there has been no public means available to verify reality, when the floodgates of traumatic memory are opened, what path should be taken? The road to proclamation of truth, and its iterations, is not a clearly marked path.

A feeling of helplessness is central to the torture cycle, according to Metin Besoglu, one of the world's leading experts on the subject of torture and mass violence trauma.[9] This helplessness is much more dramatic in a

6 President Barack Obama, White House Press Conference, 1 August 2014 (https://www.whitehouse.gov/the-press-office/2014/08/01/press-conference-president).

7 Gillian Slovo, 'Truth and Reconciliation?' *Trauma and Attachment*, eds. S. Benamer and K. White (London: Karnac Publishers, 2008), 15.

8 Inger Agger and S. B. Jensen, *Trauma and Healing under State Terrorism* (London: Zed Books, 1996), 203.

9 Metin Besoglu, *A Mental Health Care Model for Mass Trauma Survivors: Control-Focused Behavioural Treatment of Earthquake, War, and Torture* (Cambridge: Cambridge University Press, 2011).

situation where an individual knows s/he is facing an all-powerful enemy such as the state or a terror regime. So the demand for justice is problematic when it involves the state. Those who have been rendered powerless can magnify the extent of state power or, conversely, minimize the difficulty of engaging it.

The three elements of psychosocial trauma conceptualized by Martin-Baro play significant roles as individuals, families, and societies attempt to *de-privatize* the experiences of state violence. Organized violence, institutionalized lies, and social polarization each require appropriate methods to mitigate their traumatic legacy. Although each individual affected by state violence bears a wound, and likely feels helpless in the face of impunity, the cause of the injury lies in the social application of violence. Failure to address these injuries socially will undermine efforts to forge stable democratic societies when trauma and the consequences of trauma lie dormant beneath the surface of superficially created and fragile political structures.

Brazilian psychoanalyst and social critic, Jurandir Freire Costa, maintains that false or incomplete transitions lead people to a generalized state of insanity especially in societies where the politicians are cynical and opportunist.[10] Impunity, in states where past perpetrators walk freely and often continue to hold political sway, creates conditions that fail to address the effects of cognitive dissonance created by institutional lies. Issues affecting social polarization are not addressed in fear of aggravating contested memories and views of the past. While the practice of organized violence, e.g. torture, may be officially discontinued or lessened during periods of transition, its effects linger and may be aggravated by generalized denial, lack of acknowledgement, or diminishment of the phenomenon.

Chilean psychologist Elizabeth Lira developed treatment methods to assist victims of political repression under the Pinochet dictatorship.[11] While Lira looks to the past for the roots of present day problems, she also identifies current structures and policies as generating new political and social divides. The contexts in which transition societies emerge affect prospects for democratic development and social stability. Therefore, the growth of violent crime in Chile may be a shared result of the legacy of the Pinochet dictatorship, as well as the divide between haves and have-nots in a new consumer driven culture. And thus we witness how past and present can collide to influence the future.

10 Jurandir Freire Costa, 'Transcendencia e Violencia,' *Dialogos em Psicologia Social eds.* Anamaria Vilela e L. Sato (Sao Paulo: *Centro Edelstein de Pesquisas Sociais*, 2012).

11 Elizabeth Lira Kornfeld, Germán Morales Farías, eds., *Derechos humanos y Reparación: Una Discusión Pendiente* (Santiago: LOM Ediciones, Universidad Alberto Hurtado, 2005).

Sola Sierra, President of Chile's Association of Relatives of the Disappeared, spoke of the abiding impact of state violence in her last interview before her death in July 1999.

> This country lost some very fundamental values such as ethics, dignity, the ability to be shocked and substituted them with half-truths, lies, two faced attitudes, impunity and indifference toward corruption and individualism. All of this is validated by impunity, which is why truth and justice are so important as standards, not only for the families of the victims, but also because no society can establish solid moral pillars under those conditions. The truth must come out and it must be held up so that these things can never happen again.[12]

But how justice issues can be comprehensively addressed, or even construed, remains difficult to fathom in both concept and application. In the latter years of many transition governments, examples of such efforts can be identified. Truth Commissions have issued reports, trials of perpetrators have taken place, commemorative practices enacted, memorials to victims built, and economic compensation programs have been implemented. Achieved with various degrees of success, these restorative projects gesture to the significance of institutionally based responses to past state-sanctioned human rights crimes.

Dr. Yaya de Andrade, a psychologist who founded the Vancouver Association for Survivors of Torture (VAST), created numerous *circles of support* as antidotes to constructed circles of silence through her work with survivors of torture and refugees.[13] Her therapeutic interventions were founded on the conviction that culture, along with individual and collective understanding of the social context of the trauma, comprises an intrinsic consideration for treatment. An understanding of the context in which the trauma was created is fundamental to treatment. Dr. de Andrade practices a treatment model in which the meaning of the experience is pursued for both the individual survivors and the communities in which they live. The creation of circles of support entails working within networks and developing ever-expanding means of assistance and knowledge in the larger community. Schools, social service agencies, service providers, state health and welfare bureaucracies, and faith groups all play their own roles within these circles.

---

12 *Santiago Times*, July 30, 1999, viewed 23 May 2016 (website no longer valid), http://www.tcgnews.com/santiagotimes/index.php.

13 Yaya De Andrade, 'The Psychocultural Context of Trauma: Understanding Experiences of Émigré Children,' *Estudos de Psicologia* 1 (1996): 36–49.

Working in VAST and in the Toronto based Canadian Centre for Victims of Torture (CCVT), we sought models of care, not cure, and learned from the work derived from the Holocaust. In 1963, Henry Krystal, himself a survivor, performed psychiatric evaluations for Holocaust survivors in attempts to secure restitution from the West German government. His 1980 follow-up study identified the problematics of traditional treatment with this particular group. He concluded, 'the psychotherapy for posttraumatic states encountered special difficulty' in that his patients were unable to reconcile their past experience 'as having been *justified by its causes*.'[14] He found that the price for survival for many of his patients was paid by their constant witnessing and unrelenting denunciation of the Nazi regime. Krystal's insight identified the essential nature of the relationship between private pain and public accountability.

We looked to countries where the trauma had originated for the purpose of conceiving culturally relevant treatment for refugee survivors. And through our collaborative work in Brazil and Chile, we found that transitions taking place in those contexts produced new sets of complex challenges for democratic projects. It becomes essential to reflect upon the work of educators such as Paulo Freire who coined the importance of *critical consciousness* for the development of an egalitarian society in which people's voices will be heard.[15] Efforts to create opportunities and forging new values and systems assists in making connections and in (re)creating community. For those who have been directly impacted by torture, accessible and culturally appropriate treatment services are required. The assessment and understanding of psychosocial features such as existing social support and cultural beliefs in the provision of service facilitates the integration of traumatic experiences.

5 Memory and Meaning

During the two decade long Pinochet dictatorship in Chile, health professionals organized clandestinely to provide assistance to persons who had been violently repressed. FASIC, under the protection of Chilean Protestant churches, the Roman Catholic Vicariate of Solidarity, CINTRAS, and CODEPO all provided psychological support to ameliorate the traumatic consequences of torture. The basis of the therapy was the recording of individuals' repressive

14 Krystal Henry, 'Trauma and Aging,' *Trauma: Explorations in Memory*, ed. Cathy Caruth (Baltimore: The Johns Hopkins University Press, 1995), 83.

15 Paulo Freire, *Education for Critical Consciousness* (New York: Continuum Press, 1990).

experiences in efforts to provide meaning to the trauma. General Pinochet's 1998 indictment and arrest for human rights crimes was based on the compilation of thousands of these testimonies that were able to provide a strong material evidential base in support of the prosecution.

As in Chile, Brazilian psychologists are engaged in projects of memory and meaning regarding the authoritarian regime of 1964 to 1985, the violent conflicts, the horror and fear inflicted on the population, and its long-term impact on individuals, families, communities, and society at large.

A prize awarded to projects on the subject of the Civil Military Dictatorship is coordinated by the CFP (Federal Council of Psychology) and the CNDH (The National Commission of Human Rights). Psychologists continue to reflect upon the impact of the dictatorship on the psychology profession in Brazil as a way to trace memory and insert the past into the present. The group Tortura Never Again and magazines such as *Radice*, produced by psychologists from 1976 to 1981, were important to a generation of professionals working with individuals and children of those who were subjected to torture, to prison, to inhuman treatment. Testimonies by survivors continue to generate discussions and suggest methods to recover parts of a history usually dissociated from the contemporary problems of the Brazilian society.

In 2013, the profession of psychology celebrated its fifty-year anniversary in Brazil. The Paulo Freire Space, designed as a manifestation of culture, poetry, and the use of dialogue as a human rights connector, was one among many exhibits in a national conference. During the same conference a video on Vladimir Herzog, a Brazilian journalist who died in prison during dictatorship, was viewed as part of the program. These are two examples of how the practice of psychology in Brazil has evolved and an indication of what has yet to be done in a country still filled with violence, violations, corruption, and social disparity.

Other projects are emerging with the intent to make the past more known, to acknowledge those who suffered, and to seek justice by indicting those who tortured. A project entitled Psychology and the Right to Memory and Truth was conducted by the National Committee of Human Rights of the Federal Council of Psychology and it produced a valuable report in an attempt to repair the lives of those affected by the dictatorship.

Lamentably, state-organized commemorative practices have their own political limitations and, as such, often can fail to dislodge traumatic memory. There continues to be pressure from civil society organizations for the creation of committees, the recognition of human rights crimes, services, and models of care that address the larger traumatic context.

But serious barriers to the realization of truth claims and calls for justice exist. Judith Herman in her 1992 ground-breaking text, *Trauma and Recovery*, details the inherent obstacles when dealing with trauma. She gives insight into the difficulties of comprehending the precipitating origins of trauma and why these are often avoided.

> To study psychological trauma is to come face to face both with human vulnerability in the natural world and with the capacity for evil in human nature. To study psychological trauma means bearing witness to horrible events. When the events are natural disasters or "Acts of God," those who bear witness sympathize readily with the victim. But when the traumatic events are of human design, those who bear witness are caught in the conflict between victim and perpetrator. It is morally impossible to remain neutral in this conflict. The bystander is forced to take sides.[16]

Therefore, exhortations for memory, truth, and justice are not enough. The avoidance of 'the capacity for evil in human nature' and reluctance 'to bear witness' are powerful impediments to accomplishing the same. Creating incrementally wider circles of social support holds the possibility to overcome, or at least mitigate, these obstacles. Human rights campaigns and public education can assist to sensitize the public to trauma and its impact. And they can help rebuild communities that have been rent by fear and prolonged exposure to repression.

The management of trauma has implications and interdisciplinary applications. Global politics and postcolonial economies have resulted in new inequalities and political tensions, often associated with large-scale migration of populations towards North America, Australia, New Zealand, and Europe.

Treatment centres in Europe, Canada and the United States were first formed in the 1970s and 1980s to address the traumatic sequelae of survivors who managed to find asylum. Today more than 140 treatment centres across the continents belong to the International Rehabilitation Council for Torture Victims and Toronto's CCVT has assisted 19,000 survivors from 136 countries in its thirty years of service.[17] These numbers stand as a dismal testament to the condition of contemporary human rights.

---

16 Judith Herman, *Trauma and Recovery* (New York: Basic Books, 1997), 7.

17 'Report on Canada's Compliance with the Human Rights Instruments for the Occasion of the May 2013, Periodic Review of Canada,' *United Nations Human Rights: Office of the High Commissioner, OHCHR.org*, viewed 17 May 2016, http://lib.ohchr.org/HRBodies/UPR/Documents/Session16/CA/CCVT_UPR_CAN_S16_2013_%20CanadianCentreforVictimsofTorture_E.pdf.

When torture treatment centres were being established in response to the needs of newly arrived refugees in Copenhagen, Toronto, Vancouver, Los Angeles, and Minnesota, among others, one hurdle to be surmounted was to overcome the generally held notion that torture was a historic practice, rarely, if ever, occurring in the contemporary world. It was viewed apart from modernity and seemingly not extant in numbers high enough to require specialized treatment centres. Amnesty International's significant volume, *Torture in the 80s*, provided a closer reading of the reality. Indeed, evidence of torture was found to be so rampant, that the report named torture as the twentieth century epidemic. Even so, in my time as executive director of CCVT, calls would come from people who mistakenly thought the Centre for Victims of Torture was an animal rights organization since they would insist that animals are torture victims; people no longer are. Because governments that practiced torture went to great lengths to deny and hide their deeds, evidence was obscured, thus rendering torture a topic easily averted by bystanders.

Refugees escaping from traumatic experiences such as torture posed challenges for health providers. Survival mechanisms employed by individuals during flight and when seeking asylum can become impediments to resettlement and to successful refugee claims. Disassociation under conditions of imprisonment may have assisted to cope with daily horror but can pose serious problems when continued in a new context. Vigilance during escape may have assured safety but when experienced as insomnia and hyper-vigilance, can cause sleep deprivation. Suspicion of strangers may have provided protection from danger but can disrupt the forging of new relationships and networks necessary for efficacious adaptation in a new community.

The consequences for survivors can be compounded by failure of service providers to recognize traumatic consequences. Consequences are further aggravated when the host society fails to recognize the conditions in countries of origin that prompted flight. For individuals attempting to gain asylum, traumatic forgetting most certainly can derail their claims when details have been submerged in the miasma of memory. Refugee policies that position the claimant in an adversarial position where their history is subject to prosecutorial imperative provoke retraumatization. When the traumatic experience is individualized and decontextualized, circles of silence continue to follow the survivor and perpetuate isolation. Without understanding of the country conditions that prompted flight, each individual refugee claim remains subject to denial and their ordeals are kept privatized.

Multiple issues are implicated in public policy initiatives that serve to create circles of support. Importantly, humane refugee asylum regulations that recognize the context of the experience can prevent retraumatization. Deleterious detention policies that can trigger memories of prison and seem to replicate persecution negate the potential for a safe haven. Further, migration regulations that prolong family separation, or deny reunification, upset adjustment and aggravate survival guilt.

After a successful asylum claim, when the refugee flight sequence is concluded, opportunity exists to begin to re-establish disrupted life. Settlement policies that assist with finding employment, learning a new language, and provide access to social services, and health care ease adaptation. Conversely, when service is restricted, it reawakens memories of ostracism and exclusion and reinforces isolation. Conditions met in countries of asylum, most notably racism and anti-refugee sentiment, add to the pre-existing trauma and create new complications. Morton Beiser's study *Strangers at the Gate: the 'Boat People's' First Ten Years in Canada*, concludes that a singular contribution for successful settlement is the 'warmth of the welcome.'[18] The context in which survivors take up the challenges of adjustment to the new community is a critical factor for success. How refugees are received and perceived by the larger society can exacerbate or accelerate the settlement process. Public recognition of human rights crimes and their impact on individuals are essential components of circles of support and have the capacity to limit occasions that could cause retraumatization.[19]

Public policy on human rights is equally important to governmental positions on refugee admission. Revelations that countries of asylum engage in rendition leading to torture, or even pronounce support for the practice, destabilize tentative efforts at resettlement and recovery and erode the possibility for safe haven. Conversely, governmental positions on justice and impunity contribute to build environments where trauma can be alleviated. Justice alone may not heal but it does set the foundation for it. Efforts of those working for social and legal reparation have the capacity to create feelings of security and constitute a public gesture on the side of victims. They serve to make meaning of violation when there are consequences for the traumatizing events. The U.S. based Centre for Justice and Accountability, England's Redress, and the Canadian Centre for International Justice are examples of organizations working to broaden legal and educational campaigns about these human

18 Morton Beiser, *Strangers at the Gate: The 'Boat People's' First Ten Years in Canada* (Toronto: University of Toronto Press, 1999), 185.

19 Joan Simalchik, 'The Politics of Torture: Dispelling the Myths and Understanding Survivors,' *Community Support for Survivors of Torture: A Manual*, ed. K. Price (Toronto: CCVT Publications, 1995).

rights issues. They have served to sensitize lawyers, law schools, and the legal establishment to the need for victims' cases to be heard and supported, and in doing so, animated and expanded a conversation about trauma and its public policy implications.

The 1960, Adolf Eichmann trial in Israel provided Holocaust survivors with an opportunity to share their histories in the service of justice and to create a context in which they could be understood. Similar reactions occurred in the wake of the 1998 arrest of Chile's General Pinochet in Great Britain. Shattering the illusion of impunity, his victims' testimonies served as the basis of his indictment. Afterward, as in the case of Eichmann, more victims came forward for treatment in the belief that there would be a greater capacity for understanding their experiences and that they would be believed.

Countries continue to come to terms with their pasts. In August 2014, Cambodia's Extraordinary Chambers in the Courts convicted two top leaders for crimes against humanity and sentenced them to life in prison. The Court went beyond its legal jurisdiction to endorse a number of memorial initiatives to commemorate the country's 1975–79 Genocide. Proposals for a National Remembrance Day, creation of a museum and school curricular material also includes plans for a testimonial therapy project.

6 Final Remarks

The tortured past casts a long shadow and intrudes into the contemporary socio-political arena. The two main contenders in Chile's presidential election held November 2013 were women, with former President Michelle Bachelet being elected to a new term of office. Her opponent, former Senator Evelyn Matthei, is the daughter of Air Force General Fernando Matthei, a member of Pinochet's junta and government throughout the dictatorship period. Bachelet's father, Alberto, was also an Air Force General. But in his case, because he opposed the military coup d'état, he was arrested, imprisoned, and died due to complications from torture. Contended pasts leave much space for individual, community, and social intervention.

Both President Bachelet and Brazil's President Dilma Rousseff were political prisoners who survived torture and because of their experiences, they simultaneously embody the past trauma and contemporary resilience. The countries they govern today emerged from dictatorship into the new terrain of a globalized neoliberal world. The East-West divide of First and Second Worlds has been eclipsed while the formerly labelled Third World has been recast as the Global South. Structural impediments pose new challenges for eradicating social and economic polarization and organized violence.

In large urban centres in Brazil people continue to describe their reality as one impossible to change. Nevertheless, silence has been broken in many fronts. For example, women in Brazil have demanded to be heard and that actions be taken to deter violence and abuse. In 1985, the first WPD (Women's Police Department) was created and the 2006 Maria da Penha Act outlawing violence against women improved the daily domestic routine of many women and children. According to a 2005 United Nations' report:

> In 1993, there were already 125 WPD s in the country, and they filed 123,131 complaints over that one-year period. In 1999, the country had 307 WPD s and, in a study including 267 of these, a total of 411,213 offense notifications were registered that year. Only 6% of these records were transformed into inquiries instituted and/or referred to the judicial authorities. The majority of the complaints were referred to conciliation or mediation services by the WPD itself. In 2003, there were 425,935 occurrences of offenses, recorded by 289 WPD s studied. At that time, there was a total of 340 WPD s in existence.[20]

Violence and violations continue not only in domestic contexts but also in communities and government controlled areas such as jails. Scores of people are daily injured when police officers use teargas and rubber bullets to disperse demonstrators. In its 2009 report on the use of lethal force, Human Rights Watch documented how legitimate efforts to curb violent crime in São Paulo and Rio de Janeiro were undercut by police who engaged in unlawful violence and investigators who routinely failed to conduct proper inquiries into shootings by the police. José Miguel Vivanco, Americas Director at Human Rights Watch, reported that even though 'authorities have an obligation to re-establish order when violence erupts during public protests that doesn't give security forces license to violate protesters' or bystanders' rights or make them immune from punishment when they go too far.'[21]

---

20 United Nations Division for the Advancement of Women Expert Group Meeting, *Violence against Women in Brazil* (Geneva: United Nations Publications, 2005), viewed 23 May 2016, http://www.un.org/womenwatch/daw/egm/vaw-stat-2005/docs/expert-papers/d_Oliveira.pdf.

21 Human Rights Watch, *Report on Lethal Force* (New York: Human Rights Watch Publications, 2009), viewed 23 May 2016, https://www.hrw.org/report/2009/12/08/lethal-force/police-violence-and-public-security-rio-de-janeiro-and-sao-paulo.

In closing, the exercise of torture may no longer be considered epidemic in these countries, but it still remains a practice in particular contexts. All levels of government and the public in countries such as Chile and Brazil must carefully consider its impact. Current efforts to interrupt the traumatic legacy of the past can be advanced and expanded in cooperation with human rights groups. Similarly, countries providing asylum to survivors of officially created cruelties have responsibilities to act. The need for individual services for victims remains but the recognition of the long-term impact of psychosocial trauma and destruction necessitates broader social interventions such as justice initiatives, memorials and commemorative practices. Practitioners and caregivers need to recognize the historical context of individual experience and incorporate treatment practices that address these larger social sequelae. Circles of silence that surround trauma and its impact can be remedied for individuals, their families, and communities. While the trauma will not be erased, de-privatizing the experience through social and public interventions can promote amelioration.

Bibliography

Agger, Inger and S. B. Jensen. *Trauma and Healing under State Terrorism*. London: Zed Books, 1996.

Amnesty International. *Torture in the Eighties*. London: AI Publications, 1984.

Arns, Paulo. *Brazil: Never Again*. Sao Paulo: Archdiocese of Sao Paulo, 1985.

Besoglu, Metin. *A Mental Health Care Model for Mass Trauma Survivors: Control-Focused Behavioural Treatment of Earthquake, War, and Torture.* Cambridge: Cambridge University Press, 2011.

Bilbija, Ksenija and Leigh A. Payne, eds. *Accounting for Violence: Marketing Memory in Latin America*. Durham: Duke University Press, 2011.

Beiser, Morton. *Strangers at the Gate: The 'Boat People's' First Ten Years in Canada*. Toronto: University of Toronto Press, 1999.

Brewin, Andrew, Louis Duclos and David MacDonald. *One Gigantic Prison: The Report of the Fact-Finding Mission to Chile, Argentina and Uruguay*. Toronto: Inter-Church Committee on Chile, 1976.

Carinci, A. J., P. Mehta and P. J. Christo. 'Chronic Pain in Torture Victims.' *Current Pain and Headache Reports* 14.2 (2010): 73–79.

Caruth, Cathy. *Trauma: Explorations in Memory*. Baltimore: The Johns Hopkins University Press, 1995.

Carrington, Karin and Susan Griffin. *Transforming Terror: Remembering the Soul of the World*. Berkeley: University of California Press, 2011.

Collins, Cath, K. Hite and A. Joignant, eds. *The Politics of Memory in Chile: From Pinochet to Bachelet*. Boulder: First Forum Press, 2013.

De Andrade, Yaya. 'The Psychocultural Context of Trauma: Understanding Experiences of Émigré Children.' *Estudos de Psicologia* 1 (1996): 36–49.

Dorfman, Ariel. *Exorcising Terror: The Incredible Unending Trial of General Augusto Pinochet*. New York: Seven Stories Press, 2002.

Freire Costa, Jurandir. 'Transcendencia e Violencia.' *Dialogos em Psicologia Social*, edited by Anamaria Vilela and L. Sato, 87–102. Sao Paulo: Centro Edelstein de Pesquisas Sociais, 2012.

Freire, Paulo. *Education for Critical Consciousness*. New York: Continuum Press, 1990.

Herman, Judith Lewis. *Trauma and Recovery*. New York: Basic Books, 1997.

Human Rights Watch. *Report on Lethal Force*. New York: Human Rights Watch Publications, 2009.

Inter-Church Committee on Chile. *One Gigantic Prison: A Report of the Fact-finding Mission to Chile, Argentina and Uruguay*. Toronto: Canadian Council of Churches, 1976.

Krystal, Henry. 'Trauma and Aging.' *Trauma: Explorations in Memory*, edited by Cathy Caruth, 76–99. Baltimore: The Johns Hopkins University Press, 1995.

Lechner, Norbert. *Fear at the Edge: State, Terror and Resistance in Latin America*, edited by Juan Corradi, Patricia Weiss Fagen, Manuel Antonio Garreton. Berkeley: University of Berkeley Press, 1992.

Lira Kornfeld, Elizabeth and Germán Morales Farías, eds. *Derechos Humanos y Reparación: Una Discusión Pendiente*. Santiago: LOM Ediciones, Universidad Alberto Hurtado, 2005.

Martín-Baró, Ignacio, Adrianne Aron and Shawn Corne, eds. *Writings for a Liberation Psychology*. Cambridge: Harvard University Press, 1994.

O'Donnell, Guillermo. 'La Cosecha del Miedo.' *Nexos* 6.6, Mexico City, 1983.

Portello, M. E. *Displaced Memories: The Poetics of Trauma in Argentine Women's Writing*. Lewisburg: Bucknell University Press, 2009.

Rothschild, Babette. *The Body Remembers: The Psychophysiology of Trauma and Trauma Treatment*. New York: W.W. Norton, 2000.

Simalchik, Joan. 'The Politics of Torture: Dispelling the Myths and Understanding Survivors.' *Community Support for Survivors of Torture: A Manual*, edited by Kathy Price, 1–5. Toronto: CCVT Publications, 1995.

Slovo, Gillian. 'Truth and Reconciliation?' *Trauma and Attachment*, edited by S. Benamer and K. White, 11–27. London: Karnac Books, 2008.

United Nations Division for the Advancement of Women Expert Group Meeting. *Violence against Women in Brazil*. Geneva: United Nations Publications, 2005.

Volkan, Vamik and J. C. Fowler. 'Large-Group Narcissism and Political Leaders.' *A Special Issue of Psychiatric Annals*, edited by Otto Kernberg. Viewed 23 May 2016. http://www.vamikvolkan.com/large-group-narcissism-and-political-leaders.

CHAPTER 7

Unpacking Male Sexualized Trauma: Rights and Resistance from a Feminist Perspective

Anka D. Mason

Abstract

Male survivors of rape and other sexualized trauma in conflict and post-conflict communities around the world are stepping forward to end the stigmatization, isolation, shame, and silence around their victimization. As they do so, socially constructed taboos and mistaken awareness around male victimization are challenged. By framing their trauma alongside the language of rights, this chapter addresses the lacuna in knowledge and practical application of rights-based frameworks and the consequent harm and re-victimization that arise as a result. Importantly, I demonstrate how the trauma-to-rights path for male survivors of conflict-related sexual violence upends: (1) fabricated notions of the impossibility of male victimization; (2) the positioning of males as perpetrators only; and (3) global conventional standards of masculine behaviour, practices, and expression that strongly discourage any or all indications of vulnerability. I use the common threads of trauma, resistance, and rights in the works of Tarja Väyrynen (War and Trauma in Finland), Muneer Ahmad (Rights and the Dehumanization of Guantânamo Detainees), and Chris Dolan (Male Rape Survivors within the Ugandan Refugee Population) to reveal how traumatic experiences in the male body tell a story, as Arthur Frank describes, 'in order to construct new maps and new perceptions of their relationships to the world.' Observing, as some have, that the specific issue of male sexualized trauma is also a feminist one, I argue that these 'new maps' and 'new perceptions' implicate and urge the development of a new feminist discourse on gender, power, violence, and rights. This emerging discourse must in turn, effectively interrupt and resist the antiquated dichotomy of 'female/victim' and 'male/perpetrator' in order for the global community to actualize a more just application of mechanisms aimed at protecting the fundamental human rights of all persons.

Keywords

corporeity – feminism – intersubjectivity – male survivors – rape – sexual violence – trauma – rights

 | DOI:10.1163/9789004397576_009

1 Introduction

Rape and other forms of sexual violence enacted on male corporeity in conflict and post conflict communities implicate negative perceptions and cognitions of the feminine as part of the torture and humiliation of men. Male survivors become the 'unthinkable, unspeakable feminine.' Such characterizations codify the female form as the *right form* for this category of violent aggression while attackers act explicitly to 'take away their victims' masculinity. Moreover, the dominant discourse regarding conflict related sexual violence tends toward binary, narrow viewpoints of victims and perpetrators.[1] These points of view produce narratives that privilege certain types of violence and certain types of victims over others.[2] The end result is erasure of and resistance to those survivors and victims whose experiences conflict with well recognized, accepted, and elevated narratives. Thus, locating the roots of discourse narratives that support discrimination between types of harm and victims is valuable toward explaining and understanding the shared difficulties around addressing male sexualized trauma in conflict and other settings.

As a starting point, this chapter takes aim at the mechanisms that support acceptance of certain forms of traumatic violence upon the male form. Importantly, I underscore how violence through munitions and torture has been and is currently negotiated and normalized under treaties and memoranda of law by States. I then compare and contrast this acceptance of normalized conflict violence to the rejection of and resistance to narratives of male survivors of sexualized violence. This exposition reveals startling contradictions concerning how the male body is perceived, cognized, and treated when harmed within the context of armed conflict. I conclude by suggesting that only by admitting to and accepting the traumatic vulnerability of both men and women within the context of armed conflict settings can we arrive at new perceptions and consciousness regarding the trauma-to-rights path for male survivors of sexualized violence in all contexts.

Though the subject matter of this work is quite complex, the reasons for producing this writing are simple. This writing is itself a meditation on our position of choiceless-ness regarding the form we take in terms of sexed, raced, nationalized bodies at birth. We enter the world as embodied consciousness and free

1 Augusta DelZotto and Adam Jones, *Male on Male Sexual Violence: Human Rights Last Taboo* (paper presented to the Annual Convention of the International Studies Association-ISANew Orleans, LA, 23–27 March 2002), viewed 10 June 2016, http://adamjones.freeservers.com/malerape.htm.

2 Ibid.

will within a corporeal shell that is labelled, circumscribed, and constrained by family relations, communal/ethnic connections and numerous other identities. Birth and body are geopolitically and legally concretized through civil registrations processes and other bureaucratic mechanisms for creating, maintaining, and controlling the elements that make up the web of nation. Across borders and time zones, however, the harm of conflict related trauma and violence and the erasure of suffering remain ever present. This modest work aims to enhance and clarify our understanding of humanitarian principles as we strive to overcome our individual and collective tendencies toward divisionary, dichotomous, and binary expressions that erase our interconnectedness and interrelatedness.

2 Three Lenses and the Trilogy of Trauma on Male Forms

The works of Tarja Väyrynen, Muneer Ahmad, and Chris Dolan[3] present a trilogy of trauma through which I outline perceptions of harm to male forms as enacted through munitions, torture, and sexualized trauma. The trilogy illustrates some of the ways in which such violence is differentiated, experienced, perpetrated, understood and misunderstood in connection with male bodies. First, in order to reconcile the role that shared perspectives play, I incorporate the lens of *intersubjectivity* into this analysis. Here, it denotes

> that meeting of minds by which two [or more] selves take each other's meaning (here, "feminization" and "dehumanization") with reference to the same object (here, sexualized and other forms of violence enacted upon the bodies of men) beheld in common.[4]

Intersubjectivity is also examined within the context of 'figured worlds'[5] of nation and national identity created and maintained through collective and integrated activities within the social realm.[6] Critically examining the ways nation emerges from a collective construct and then controls, develops, and frames dominant discourses on gender and gendered performance is an

3 Chris Dolan is herein used to denote the collective work of the Uganda Refugee Law Project under the direction of Dr. Chris Dolan.

4 Walker Percy, 'Symbol, Consciousness and Intersubjectivity,' *The Journal of Philosophy* 55.15 (July 1958): 631.

5 Helen Ting, 'Social Construction of Nation: A Theoretical Exploration,' *Nationalism and Ethnic Politics* 467 (2008): 453–482, viewed 21 July 2014, doi: 10.1080/13537110802301418.

6 Ibid.

important piece to the puzzle for unpacking reactions surrounding sexualized trauma in males of conflict communities.

I employ corporeity, as formulated by Maurice Merleau-Ponty, as the second lens. His supposition that 'the body is our general means of having a world,'[7] is most useful in emphasizing the importance of considering how ideological and gendered constructions inform and shape ideas around rights as connected with the human body. I recognize and agree with the viewpoint of human rights as contested claims contextualized by 'material existence'[8] that are further situated around modes of production and reproduction.[9] Herein, however, rights contestation is also complicated by the male/female binary as related to competing notions of protection and destruction.

Finally, the third lens, the feminist perspective, endorses a relational view of beliefs and practices anchored in contesting the use of corporeity as bases for denial of rights and equality. This part of the examination considers Catharine A. MacKinnon's declaration of how '[b]eing a woman is not yet a name for a way of being a human being.'[10] It is this *dehumanized femaleness* that I contend supports the constructions of the 'feminization of victimization' and the 'masculinization of oppression'[11] with respect to sexual violence against males. Through this lens we locate purposeful and violent subjugation of male bodies as part of a patriarchal repertoire for maintaining 'social structures' of power.[12] Thus, we capture within our sights patriarchy against males, and this provides space for considering how and why resistance to *seeing as traumatic* violence and especially sexualized violence against male corporeity, is so pervasive.

---

7 Taylor Carman, 'The Body in Husserl & Merleau-Ponty,' *Philosophical Topics* 27.2 (1999): 214.

8 Gary Teeple, *The Riddle of Human Rights* (New York: Humanity Books, 2005), 21.

9 Ibid., 22–31.

10 Carol Rittner, 'Are Women Human?' *Rape: Weapon of War and Genocide*, ed. Carol Rittner and John K. Roth (St. Paul: Paragon House, 2012), 3.

11 Andy Fisher, Rick Goodwin and Mark Patton, *Men and Healing: Theory, Research, and Practice in Working with Male Survivors of Childhood Sexual Abuse,*(Ottawa: The Men's Project, 2009), 14.

12 Sylvia Walby, 'Theorising Patriarchy,' *Sociology* 23.2 (May 1989): 214. Walby's definition of patriarchy as social structure is useful in considering male sexualized trauma and gendering issues as she argues that '[t]he use of the term social structure ... clearly implies rejection of both biological determinism and the notion that every individual man is in a dominant position and every individual woman in a subordinate one.' Quote also found on page 14, viewed 10 June 2015, http://www.opensocietyfoundations.org/voices/after-more-decade-truth-about-cia-torture-poland?utm_source=justice_B&utm_medium=e-mail&utm_content=I7z LaWOhOGYXvqdozQ_MUQRp3i3P5eePKJB7Qe40-gc&utm_campaign=j ustice_B_072514.

In considering the trauma of the male rape survivors, we who are the children of societies built on patriarchal oppression, dominance, and violence in service of power, face a stunning reversal of formal and informal representations of violence. We who manifest phenomenologically as women face complex emotions, ideas, and reactions based on broad and sweeping personal and collective histories of oppression, sexism, enslavement, and the historical through present day environments of sexual trauma, as we consider male survivor experiences of sexual violence. To complicate matters further, both women and men face the unimaginably degrading and yet prevalent ideology that the male rape victim is *made into a woman* after being rape. Women's bodies, experiences, and existences, are erased with this pronouncement and in this instance, we are made into the objectified, stigmatizing tool of violent male oppression against other males. The thinking goes something like this: to have a male enter you is to be in the subordinate position, which is the position that is *rightfully* female. Thus, to enter a male is to subordinate him and *make him a woman.* This positioning is the language of domination and thus carries with it all of the overtones of power relations within societies built around violent, hegemonic patriarchal practices. All women's power is obliterated. Being a woman and *being made into a woman* become the markers of weakness and grave suffering. And yet, all humans brought into being, brought into life, must travel through the bodies of women to exist, this includes all men. It is the woman's body that is ruptured, cut open, and at times placed at grave risk of death, to bring the human baby forth to draw its first breath. Women bear the pain and discomfort of months of nurturing the human foetus, and when at last the baby is due, woman, with all the force within her, renders forth a child into the world. At this point the woman is at her most vulnerable *and* most powerful, for she is literally giving life, pushing life into the world. In the violently twisted mind of a rapist, this is of no importance.

In the minds of those insisting on the use of rape and sexual violence as a weapon of war, men and women are implicated equally. Agents of powerful nation-states and their allies often act with impunity, using threats of sexual violence as part of the violent subjugation of men, as demonstrated in the findings of fact in *Al-Nashiri v. Poland*, where the European Court of Human Rights addressed the CIA's use of torture against Abd al-Rahim al-Nashiri. The Court found as fact that:

> *In Poland, U.S. interrogators subjected Nashiri to mock executions with a power drill as he stood naked and hooded, racked a semi-automatic handgun close to his head as he sat shackled before them, held him in 'standing*

> *stress positions,' and* ***threatened to bring in his mother and sexually abuse her in front of him.***[13]

Here we witness nation, collectively constructed and violently defended through its agents, wielding sexual violence as a tool. Agents of nation-state play out constructions of gender, hegemonic violence, and torture in the name of national security. Male victims of rape and other forms of sexual violence in conflict settings are often subjected to various forms of violation of bodily integrity. In reporting on male survivors in Uganda, Will Stor recounts that:

> men aren't simply raped, they are forced to penetrate holes in banana trees that run with acidic sap, to sit with their genitals over a fire, to drag rocks tied to their penis, to give oral sex to queues of soldiers, to be penetrated with screwdrivers and sticks.[14]

In reading and attempting to integrate, *make-sense of*, and *find meaning* in these testimonies, we must consider our own connection with body, identity, and closeness or distance with traumatised 'other.'

Bessel A. van der Kolk posits that the work of those helping the traumatised consists of assisting victims and survivors of traumatic experiences to stay in their bodies and make sense of what they are experiencing when traumatic events resurface in the mind and manifest physically in the body.[15] How do we, as readers and witnesses, stay present within our bodies as we take in accounts by victims and survivors of sexual violence used as a weapon of war? Nation-states have answered by turning trauma into heroism, citing torture as necessary against monolithic evil, and re-purposing sexual violence as part of the repertoire of tools used to secure homelands and borders. As individuals comprising nation, we must look to the experiences of those daring to resist the re-writing of their traumas to understand the re-present and re-member these experiences in order reconcile the horror of this part of our humanity.

---

13 Amrit Singh, 'After More Than a Decade, the Truth About CIA Torture in Poland' *Open Society Justice Initiative*, 24 July 2014 (These details were corroborated in a report by the CIA's own Inspector General). Bolded emphasis author's.

14 Will Stor, 'The Rape of Men: The Darkest Secret of War,' *The Observer*, 17 July 2011.

15 Claudia Ucros, 'Approche Somatique du Psychotrauma: Un autre regard psychothérapeutique?' *Stress et Truama* 4.2 (2004): 122.

3 Heroic vs. Traumatic

War intensifies our notional corporeity. Male and female forms within armed-conflict settings take on multi-dimensional subjective and intersubjective identities. For example, under international human rights and humanitarian law, women and children are entitled to special protected status in armed conflict settings.[16] On the other hand, treaties enacted as far back as 1868 articulate norms for mutilating, wounding, and annihilating flesh and bone of male forms through the regulation of various types of munitions.[17] Further, nation-states and non-state armed groups often use public, heroic, intersubjective narratives regarding the role of male bodies, in opposition to female, young, old, and sick bodies, ignoring traumatic victimization of males, thereby completely erasing the harm or re-imagining it as useful and necessary.[18] Indeed, Tarja Väyrynen—speaking of the experiences of Finnish men and narrations of masculinity during the Finnish civil war and World War II—concludes that such intense reification of corporeity is necessary precisely because:

> Nation-states require a certain type of male bodies for warfare, and thereby in war it elevates and prioritizes some bodies and forms of hegemonic masculinity over others. From male bodies the hegemonic masculine virtues of killing and dying on behalf of the nation-state are assumed during the acts of protecting the nation, women, children, the elderly, and the infirm.[19]

The gendered and supposedly *masculine virtues of killing and dying* become a way of excusing, even selling, the prospect of the wholesale slaughter of male forms. Here Väyrynen sketches the nation-state as agent for male corporeity within its borders and its gendered performance within the theatre of war.

---

16 Articles 76–78 of the Additional Protocol I to the Geneva Conventions, of 12 August 1949 United Nations Treaty Collections, and Relating to the Protection of Victims of International Conflicts (1979) 38–40, Stating, '[w]omen shall be the object of special respect and shall be protected in particular against rape, forced prostitution and any other form of indecent assault.'

17 Declaration Renouncing the Use, in Time of War, of Explosive Projectiles Under 400 Grammes Weight. Saint Petersburg, 29 November / 11 December 1868.

18 Tarja Väyrynen, 'Keeping the Trauma of War Open in the Body: Resisting the Hegemonic Forms of Masculinity and National Identity in Visual Arts,' *Journal of Gender Studies* nv (2013): 3.

19 Ibid., 3–4.

However, such claims to corporeity and mediation of masculinity through narrative also require interconnected webs of intersubjective understanding. Indeed, Janie Leatherman observes that, 'masculinity does not exist in and of itself. *It is relational*.'[20] She elaborates further, stating, '[h]egemonic masculinity sets up oppositional masculinities through a system of power relations that affect both women and men.'[21] This assessment helps explain the creation and maintenance of subordinate and marginalized masculinities, which in turn, assists us in seeing the foundations of traumatic violence within the male experience.

We may further locate intensification of gendered corporeity, power relations, and the denial of victim status to males by observing training rituals of soldiers within combat preparatory communities. For example, in extreme circumstances, such training communities incorporate sexualized violence as a means of preparing the *certain types of male bodies* for war. Aaron Belkin demonstrates this dramatically in his examination of the use of male rape and sexual assault as initiation ritual within the ranks of the United States military late in the twentieth century. Recounting the use of forced penetration as a means of determining among other things, 'what it means to be a warrior in the US military,'[22] Belkin states:

> They forced broom handles, fingers and penises into each other's anuses. They stuck pins into flesh and bones. They vomited into one another's mouths and forced rotten foods down each other's throats. They inserted tubes into each other's anal cavities and then pumped grease through those tubes.[23]

Importantly, and in stark contrast to Belkin's subjects, when Seppo Salmenin, one of Väyrynen's artist-subjects, carves into his own body, he does so in order to generate powerful visual contestations to the re-imagining of wounds of combat as heroic.[24] In so doing, Väyrynen contends that Salmenin 'challenges the master narrative of Finnish heroism.'[25] Salmenin's art refutes the

20 Janie L. Leatherman, *Sexual Violence and Armed Conflict* (Cambridge: Polity Press, 2011), 19.

21 Ibid.

22 Aaron Belkin, *Bring Me Men: Military Masculinity and the Benign Facade of American Empire, 1898–2001* (New York: Columbia University Press, 2012), 80.

23 Ibid.

24 Väyrynen, 'Keeping the Trauma,' 10.

25 Ibid.

nation-state's appropriation of body and narrative that turned his own father into a choiceless, wounded, abstracted disposable male form.[26]

Many philosophers consider the reduction of human beings to things as one of the first forms of violence. Indeed, Simone Weil captured this sentiment effectively in her piece *Iliade ou le poème de la force*. Defining force as the *true hero* and *true subject* of this Homeric poem, she illustrates her point, stating:

> Force is what makes someone subsumed under it a thing. When it is brought to bear fully, it turns man into a thing in the most literal sense because it makes him a cadaver. Where once there was someone, a moment later, there is no one.[27]

Here we observe the resonance of Weil's observation with Salmenin's message: the reduction through force, intentionally directed toward destruction (also how many types of violence may be defined) of the human being. We are also given, by this definition, the opportunity to see the space for resistance to this reduction. That is to say, we may resist the reduction itself before it manifests in the more extreme violent dimensions toward a specified end.

Reduction itself, as an ingredient of force and violence, runs across a spectrum and is demonstrable as words, thoughts, and action externally and internally directed. In other words, we are, in many respects and at each moment, subject to reduction through the thoughts, words, and actions of both others and ourselves. In this way, we capture a key ingredient of oppression, again, external and internalized, in its nakedness. We must be careful, however, to distinguish between the activity of reduction undertaken as a means of engagement in communicative acts, and reduction undertaken with the *intentionality toward destruction*, employed and incorporated with violence as a means to maintaining dominance and power. And war brings us across the entire spectrum of reduction of existence of individuals to things.

In Väyrynen's piece on artists' protests against war through the reanimation of the body within the minds of spectators, considered under Weil's contention, what we witness is the protest against this first violence of reduction through the rendering of violent, reductivists' acts. Indeed, Salmenin's use of body *parts* and focus upon what is done to the flesh, returns us to Weil's reflections on the role of force in service of a cause *heroic* and therefore the violence of reduction. Weil considered not only the effects of violence in relation to the

26 Ibid., 1.

27 Simone Weil, *Iliade ou le poème de la force* (Marseille 1940–1941), 2, viewed 10 June 2016, http://www.ebooksgratuits.com/pdf/weil_iliade.pdf.

dead, she also urged deliberation on the reification of the living, both the purveyors and recipients of violence. The violence of traumatic reduction arrests process and progress toward knowledge of self as dynamic, as phenomenological. It creates a glacier around awareness of body as integrally linked with world and other, freezing thought in such a way as to inhibit the free movement of consciousness toward its liberation. The violence implicit in norm creation and maintenance, in the implementation of institutional processes in the control and formation of citizenry, in the suppression of dissent, in the oppression of groups within society, and of course, war, is violence of reification toward control or, as seen in the case of the Holocaust and other genocides, toward complete elimination.

Nation building and maintenance is often the aim of violence, traumatic reduction within conflict and post-conflict settings. Nation and nationalism are subjectively and intersubjectively constructed and reified through bureaucratic practices, myths, traditions, and 'structures of signification.'[28] Because nation-state itself becomes corporeal through these reification processes, it is also a site of contestation and thus, vulnerability. As such, nation-states must continually generate norms, laws, and morals, and thereby create within their borders bodies that conform to that which is seen as controlling the agency and free will of the individually gendered and sexed corps. How does nation as a rights-granting, institutional concept exist when individual bodies are harmed in these circumstances that are about nation building, national security, national stabilization? That is to say our inquiry revolves around how in the name of nation the body becomes the place of harm, even though nation can be thought of as the skin that citizens wear to protect the hypoderm of individual self, constructed within its borders from harms of others. Sadly, as shown below, when that harm is enacted on the body by those agents acting as keepers of nation, we may say that nation becomes a cancerous skin, poisoning itself and that which it usually covers, and when left unattended, eventually killing the organism it was designed to protect.

4 Tortured Rights

Whereas Väyrynen's piece considers the of appropriation of male bodies for war, traumatized and made heroic through nation-state narratives, Muneer Ahmad's piece reveals the tortured male body occupying the opposite side of

28 Ting, 'Social Construction of Nation.'

the spectrum of relational, violent and violated, masculinized embodiment. He traces the United States Government's creation of the menacing, darkened, foreign, terroristic male body and its path from enemy-combatant to Guantánamo *detainee' in the US war on terror.*[29] Far from heroic-warrior status, here the nation-state narrated traumatized male corporeity as *dehumanized.* The tortured body became condemned spectacle, purposefully confined and propelled into 'inescapably stressful event[s] that overwhelmed [its] existing coping mechanisms.'[30] Because the terroristic body in this context is conceived of and perceived as *a thing to be feared*, it is objectified out of its humanity and protection under law. As Peter Halewood states:

> Bodies are both present and absent in torture and human rights law, appearing and disappearing where convenient, e.g., the body can lose its corporeality and become characterized as a mere 'liberty interest' to be balanced against society's 'security interest.'[31]

Halewood's claim is evidenced in Ahmad's narrative regarding Omar Khader, the youngest Guantánamo prisoner and Ahmad's client for three years.[32] According to Ahmad, Khader's adolescent body was doused with solvent and used as a human mop to wipe up urine he could no longer hold after being denied a bathroom break during his interrogation.[33] Additionally, Khader's interrogators threatened him with rendition and rape by older men.[34] Speaking to the erasure of rights in relation to Khader's corporeity and torture, Ahmad states,

> What we see at Guantánamo is the inverse of citizenship: no right to have rights, a rights vacuum that enables extreme violence, so as to place Guantánamo at the centre of a struggle not merely for rights, but for humanity—that state of being that distinguishes human life from mere biological existence.[35]

29 Muneer I. Ahmad, 'Resisting Guantánamo: Rights at the Brink of Dehumanization,' *Northwestern University Law Review* 103.4 (2009): 1695–1699.

30 Bessel A. van der Kolk, 'Trauma and Memory,' *Traumatic Stress: The Effects of Overwhelming Experience on Mind, Body, and Society*, eds. Bessel A. van der Kolk, Alexander C. McFarlane and Lars Weisaeth (New York: The Guildford Press, 1996), 279.

31 Peter Halewood, 'Sameness/Difference, International Human Rights Law and the Political Meaning of Torture,' *Berkeley La Raza Law Journal* 22.1 (2012): 259.

32 Ahmad, 'Resisting Guantánamo,'1686.

33 Ibid., 1691.

34 Ibid.

35 Ibid., 1687.

Guantánamo prisoners resisted erasure through hunger strikes used to purposefully engage the state in violence (through force feeding) thereby achieving re-animation into human form and into humanity.[36] The State's reply through force-feeding necessitated acknowledgement of a *human life in being* to be saved.[37] And whereas Väyrynen's artists display wounds on the body as visual contestation to the nation-state's narrative of heroism, Guantánamo prisoners had to re-traumatize their bodies through the act of the hunger strike in order to return to the human *community*[38] and thus, ascend to rights. The prisoners' use of their corporeity in this way and the nation-state's response through force-feeding illustrates Arendt's observation that 'the strength of even the strongest individual can always be overpowered by the many who often will combine for no other purpose than to ruin strength precisely because of its peculiar independence.'[39]

We live nation as narrative enhanced through traumatic violence on the forms within borders. We pass on myths and traditions, sites of sense or meaning-making and incorporate justifications of violence. Power elites and institutional structures that utilize the traumatic impact of insider/outsider politics to further bind populations to narratives of nation and national identity. Merleau-Ponty's *body as means of having world*, folds into nation, masses of land defended through violence and laws, as means of supporting body. How are we to understand the connection between a nation's use of notions of sacrifice and scarcity to justify armed violence to control allocation of resources for all bodies that often necessitates the creation of monolithic enemy 'other'? In the US's war on terror, the masculine body of enemy other was decontextualised from humanity. Guantanamo prisoners were reduced to things and as things became disposable in the name of national security of American corporeity.

Thus here, nation-state power secured through violence of torture and used to overcome individual resistance to the removal of rights and erasure, demonstrates clearly the falsity of the impossibility of male victimization. Further, we are able to break from the fiction of males as perpetrators only and never victims by observing the creation of subordinate/marginalized male positions through violence, institutional and state terror narratives, and the erasure of rights as applied to these bodies.[40] Indeed, it is through understanding torture

---

36 Ibid., 1758–1759.

37 Ibid.

38 Ibid., 1748–1749.

39 Hannah Arendt, *On Violence* (New York: Houghton Mifflin Harcourt, 1970), 65.

40 Leatherman, *Sexual Violence*, 19–20.

as state violence perpetrated against subordinated/marginalized men that we are able to correctly capture the relationship between power and violence. With this in mind, we can then examine sexualized trauma on male forms, correcting the mistaken awareness of the myth of the impossibility of male victimization and the myth of invulnerability of the male form with respect to this type of violence.

5 Male Sexualized Trauma and Resisting Resistance

In the documentaries *They Slept with Me* and *Gender against Men*,[41] male survivors of conflict-related sexual violence in Uganda describe in detail the hours and sometimes days of repeated gang rapes, sexual violence, and humiliation.[42] They speak of rejection within medical and other care communities as well as outright denials to remedy and rights recognition as high up as the United Nations.[43] Julius Okwere, an Acholi village elder and survivor, recounts the repeated rapes he endured at the hands of government soldiers during a particular campaign of terror in April 1987.[44] His filmed testimony sets in motion resistance to resistance. The perpetrators' narratives of feminization and dehumanization lose their power of paralysis. Okwere's narrative overturns the intersubjective agreements that undergird the fictitious belief of the impossibility of male victimization.

Faced with institutional indifference, sexism, and externalized and internalized oppressive narratives, Okwere and another survivor agreed to let their recorded accounts be shown in their villages, without having their faces obscured. Resistance understood in this context of traumatic wounding to male forms is a resistance to the assigning of value, weight, and relevance to corporeity in an effort to reify it into abstraction. It is resistance to destruction of their bodies as general means of having worlds.

In viewing *They Slept with Me,* we discover narrative transcending the constructs of right-body/wrong-body for rape. Located within our own corporeity and intersubjectivity, we are challenged in our maintenance of any tendency toward re-imagining such horror as anything other than grave human

41 (Refugee Law Project, *Gender against Men* 2009) (Refugee Law Project, *They Slept with Me* 2011). A synopsis of the film *Gender against Men* is used as a lead-in to *They Slept with Me,* as the former is what gave rise to the conception and subsequent production of the latter.

42 R. L. Project 2011 *They Slept With Me.*

43 Ibid.

44 Ibid.

suffering. The survivors in the film reclaim agency of narrative and in so doing, chart alternative paths toward healing. Thus, we identify a consistency with Väyrynen's claim of the importance of keeping trauma open on the male body to resist hegemonic, hero narratives so often associated with war. Moreover, we locate the trauma narrative returning male survivors of violence from erasure toward the 'right to have rights'[45] as demonstrated in Ahmad's piece on torture at Guantánamo.

Under international law and in the name of [*weakening*] *the military forces of the enemy*,[46] nation-states may do what is necessary *to disable the greatest number of men*.[47] Treaties regulating the use of force, weapons, and protection of various populations, call on parties to weigh military necessity against superfluous and disproportionate injury.[48] At issue, however, is the fact that differing perceptions held by warring parties give rise to differing interpretations of military necessity and harm beyond limits set in treaties.[49] Far too often, civilian women, children, and men are perceived and cognized as supporting the enemy and therefore constituting *enemy forces*.[50] Under this intersubjectivity around the term *enemy forces*, rape and sexual violence are conceived of as legitimate means of *weakening the enemy*. Indeed, in *They Slept with Me*, Okwere recounts how government soldiers accused him of supporting the enemy forces prior to raping him.[51] Okwere's body became *enemy* then *dehumanized* as a lead-up to the sexual violence. Here, we are reminded of Merleau-Ponty's assertion that:

> [e]very external perception is immediately synonymous with a certain perception of [the] body, just as perception of [the] body is made explicit in the language of external perception.[52]

Thus, as applied to sexualized violence in conflict, Merleau-Ponty's assertion indicates that in war, there is no *safe*, sexed body.

---

45 Ahmad, 'Resisting Guantánamo,' 1687.

46 Declaration Renouncing the Use, in Time of War, of Explosive Projectiles Under 400 Grammes Weight. Saint Petersburg, 29 November / 11 December 1868.

47 Ibid.; See also Joshua F. Berry, 'Hollow Point Bullets: How History Has Hijacked Their Use in Combat and Why it is Time to Reexamine the 1899 Hague Declaration Concerning Expanding Bullets,' *Military Law Review* 206 (2010): 136.

48 Berry, 'Hollow Point Bullets,' 102.

49 Betcy Jose-Thota, 'The Fog of Protection: Contested Meanings and Deliberate Civilian Deaths During Armed Conflict' (Ph.D diss., University of Pittsburg, 2011), 118.

50 Ibid., 138–144.

51 *They Slept with Me*, Documentary.

52 Carmen, 'Body in Husserl' 221–222.

Since the moment of death for each sentient being is unknown, each breath places life on the threshold, squarely within the truth of liminality as the constant, permanent, and truest state of existence. The degree to which we use our free will, intentionality, and consciousness to pursue a fixed status in contradiction of liminal existence is the degree to which we suffer and cause each other harm. Simone Weil's statement of how death is what makes a human being into a thing in the most literal sense supports this. 'Killing and dying on behalf of the nation state,' as cited by Väyrynen, is yet another example. Codifying existence toward reification, through identity, national or other, is the living version of this subsistence. Conflict is an example of how traumatic liminality can produce and sustain desire to seize and anchor self to identity, place, the material so as to avoid the pain and insecurity of threshold existence. Nations exists as symbolic *imagined* worlds within liminal existence reified through the use of social structures that organize resources, power, and institutions to govern and manage the bodies within its borders. The Guantanamo prisoners exist within the violent liminality produced by the anchored, fixed State. Rape as a weapon of war is used to produce states of endless suffering, beyond physical wounds that scar over. Perpetrators seek to destroy community and familial bonds, casting into liminal space the subjective and intersubjective sense within individuals of place or security.

Nation-state's control of body through the use of *structures of meaning* is evident here where agents of nation-state use rape and sexual violence on the bodies of men and control how such violence is conceived, mediated, and understood in the broader social context. This *understanding* of sexual violence as turning *men into women*, however, was not strong enough to silence all survivors in this instant. Indeed, voices of those not living nation as majority, but rather in the margins, and thus targeted by the state's army (in this case the Acholi men) became the voices of change. Understanding symbolic, myth-making and meaning-making rapports that support the destruction of individuals and communities in the aftermath of sexual violence is important in understanding how to reverse the process. Rights discourses that exclude considerations of male victim and survivor accounts of conflict sexual violence must be challenged where those engaged in such discourses insist on narrow constructions of harm as related to certain types of bodies.

Interestingly, the trauma-to-rights path for male survivors highlights and reinvigorates the core argument that feminists have made for decades: that fundamental human rights and protections should not be abrogated based on the form of the body that is harmed. In her 1994 essay titled *Are Women Human*?, Catharine A. MacKinnon critiques the Universal Declaration of Human Rights by highlighting the ways in which women's corporeity is abused, objectified, sold, traded, and openly subject to discrimination, even as equality is proclaimed throughout the document.[53] Sexualized violence on male corporeity as discussed herein emerges here as a 'feminist issue'[54] precisely because it reveals the same absurdity regarding rights protections as equal when male victims of sexual violence face rejection based solely on the sex *and* gendering of their corporeity. Perhaps the male subjects in the works of Väyrynen, Ahmad, and Dolan could and should pose the same questions regarding their experiences around war, torture, and sexualized violence: *Is it trauma yet*? Thus, it is through answering this question that we are urged toward new understandings and responses that nullify and disconfirm harmful, gendered, and prejudicial interpretations of sexualized male trauma as well as other harm to male forms.

6 Conclusion

The trauma-to-rights path with respect to sexual violence is one that is undergoing much needed repaving and it is necessary to begin to work in a cross-disciplinary way that addresses *sexing* and *gendering* of bodies with respect to the trauma of violence within conflict communities. Rights documents at their foundation are about the security of bodies. If, however, some bodies are entitled to greater security from certain types of harm because of the form that they happen to take, then the fundamental principle of equality within rights-based documents, practices, and frameworks is lost.

Perhaps the reason that the problem of sexual violence as a weapon of war has yet to be solved is because the concept of nations has not been properly acknowledged as a construct and that nations as such are simply not capable of protecting their citizens. What is nation if it is killing its own to become something subjective and intersubjectively contested? What is nation where the bodies of other are tortured in the name of national security? What is nation when those that are raped in the process of formation or securitization, are ignored in the aftermath? Why does the trauma within nation building and securing become the problem of the individual in the aftermath? This makes sense only if nation exists as a shared imaginary space.

---

53 Carol Rittner, 'Are Women Human,' *Rape: Weapon of War and Genocide* (St. Paul: Paragon House, 2012), 1–13.

54 Lara Stemple, Interview, *Aljazeera Inside Story, The Silent Male Victims of Rape*, aired 11 July 2011 (2012 Refugee Law Project) DVD.

The solution, therefore, is to begin the arduous task of deconstructing nation, binaries of female/male, and notions of the *safer* body in conflict settings, and to address the hidden assumptions and sexist/gendered associations of trauma and harm with regard to notions of protection and destruction. We can begin our work within this suggested solution by exploring how we understand body and trauma, our notions of narrative about *self* and *other* with respect to subjective and intersubjective perceptions, and rights with respect to assignments in accordance with sexed bodies. In this way, we can reconstruct and repave the path toward a more inclusive and equal realization of rights.

The works of Väyrynen, Ahmad, and Dolan clarify the need to dismantle the constructs that privilege care responses for violence to female corporeity while ignoring the same with regard to male corporeity. Liberating ourselves from the mistaken awareness that arises as a result of false distinctions between female and male forms in connection with violence must also entail deconstructing beliefs that certain forms are acceptable targets for war, torture, and annihilation through munitions, while other forms are normalized as 'approved of' with regard to rape and sexual violence. The continued appropriation of corporeity according to sexed distinctions (or any other distinctions for that matter) for particular kinds of violence is simply unsupportable and inconsistent with aspirations of the full realization of human rights for all.

Bibliography

Ahmad, Muneer I. 'Resisting Guantánamo: Rights at the Brink of Dehumanization.' *Northwestern University Law Review* 103.4 (2009): 1683–1763.

Arendt, Hannah. *On Violence.* New York: Houghton Mifflin Harcourt, 1970.

Belkin, Aaron. *Bring Me Men: Military Masculinity and the Benign Facade of American Empire, 1898–2001.* New York: Columbia University Press, 2012.

Berry, Joshua F. 'Hollow Point Bullets: How History Has Hijacked Their Use in Combat and Why it is Time to Reexamine the 1899 Hague Declaration Concerning Expanding Bullets.' *Military Law Review* 206 (2010): 88–156.

Carmen, Taylor. 'The Body in Husserl & Merleau-Ponty.' *Philosophical Topics* 27.2 (1999): 205–226.

Cronk, George. 'James and the Problem of Intersubjectivity: An Interperative Critique.' Edited by W.R. Corti. *The Philosophy of William James* (Felix Meiner Verlag), 1976: 221–244.

DelZotto, Augusta and Adam Jones. 'Male on Male Sexual Violence in Wartime (DelZotto/ Jones).' *adamjones.freeservers.com.* August 22, 2012. Viewed January 3, 2014. http://adamjones.freeservers.com/malerape.htm.

Fisher, Andy, Rick Goodwin, with Mark Patton. *MEN & HEALING: Theory, Research, and Practice in Working with Male Survivors of Childhood Sexual Abuse.* Ottawa, ON: The Men's Project, 2009.

Halewood, Peter. 'Sameness/Difference, International Human Rights Law and the Political Meaning of Torture.' *Berkeley La Raza Law Journal* 22.1 (2012): 257–268.

International Committee of the Red Cross. 'War and Law: Treaties and State Parties to Such Treaties.' *International Committee of the Red Cross, War and Law.* January 10, 2014. Viewed 13 August 2013. http://www.icrc.org/ihl/INTRO/130?OpenDocument.

Jose-Thota, Betcy. 'The Fog of Protection: Contested Meanings and Deliberate Civilian Deaths During Armed Conflict.' PhD diss., University of Pittsburg, 2011.

Leatherman, Janie L. *Sexual Violence and Armed Conflict.* Cambridge: Polity Press, 2011.

Percy, Walker. 'Symbol, Consciousness and Intersubjectivity.' *The Journal of Philosophy* 55.15 (July 1958): 631–641.

Refugee Law Project. 'Gender Against Men.' 2009, Kampala, Uganda: RLP, DVD.

Refugee Law Project. *They Slept With Me.* 2012, Kampala, Uganda: RLP, DVD.

Refugee Law Project. Makerere University School of Law and University of California School of Law International Human Rights Clinic. 'Promoting Accountability for Conflict Related Sexual Violence Against Men: A Comparative Legal Analysis of International and Domestic Laws Relating to IDP and Refugee Men in Uganda.' *Refugee Law Project Working Paper No. 24.* Kampala, July 2013.

Rittner, Carol and John K. Roth. *Rape: Weapon of War and Genocide.* St. Paul: Paragon House, 2012.

Singh, Amrit. 'After More Than a Decade, the Truth About CIA Torture in Poland.' *Open Society Justice Initiative* 24, July 2014. Viewed 10 June 2016. http://www.opensociety-foundations.org/voices/after-more-decade-truth-about-cia-torture-poland?utm_source=justice_B&utm_medium=email&utm_content= I7zLaWOhOGYXvqdozQ_MUQRp3i3P5eePKJB7Qe40-gc&utm_campaign= justice_B_072514.

Stor, Will. 'The Rape of Men: The Darkest Secret of War,' *The Observer*, 17 July 2011. Viewed 14 February 2013. http://www.theguardian.com/society/2011/jul/17/the-rape-of-men?CMP=twt_gu

Teeple, Gary. *The Riddle of Human Rights.* Amherst, New York: Humanity Books, 2005.

Ting, Helen. 'Social Construction of Nation: A Theoretical Exploration.' *Nationalism and Ethnic Politics* 14.3 (August 14, 2008): 453–482. Viewed 21 July 2014. doi: 10.1080/13537110802301418.

Ucros, Claudia. 'Approche Somatique du Psychotrauma: un autre regard psychothérapeutique?' *Stress et Truama* 4.2 2004: 122.

van der Kolk, Bessel A. 'Trauma and Memory.' *Traumatic Stress: The Effects of Overwhelming Experience on Mind, Body, and Society*, edited by Bessel A. van der Kolk, Alexander C. McFarlane, and Lars Weisaeth, 279–302. New York: The Guildford Press, 1996.

Väyrynen, Tarja. 'Keeping the Trauma of War Open in the Body: Resisting the Hegemonic Forms of Masculinity and National Identity in Visual Arts.' *Journal of Gender Studies* nv (2013): 1–15.

Vermeulen, Maite. 'Hidden Victims: The story of sexual violence against men in armed conflict.' *e-International Relations*. September 4, 2011. Viewed 22 August 2013. http://www.e-ir.info/2011/09/04/hidden-victims-the-story-of-sexual-violence-against-men-in-armed-conflict/.

Walby, Sylvia. 'Theorising Patriarchy.' *Sociology* 23.2 (1989): 213–234.

Weil, Simone. *Iliade ou le poème de la force*. Marseille 1940–1941. Viewed 10 June 2016. http://www.ebooksgratuits.com/pdf/weil_iliade.pdf.

CHAPTER 8

Worlds after War: Negotiating the Art of Losing in J.R.R. Tolkien's *The Lord of the Rings*

Stephanie Y. Tam

Abstract

'How was it that Tolkien ... could have gone through the Great War with all of its rants and lies and still come out committed to a "feudal" literary style?'[1] Hugh Brogan's query captures the critical response of bewilderment towards the Great War veteran J.R.R. Tolkien's *The Lord of the Rings*, his fantastical epic of Middle-earth rich with medieval influences. What could the turn to fantasy and the recuperation of chivalric and out-dated convictions offer for a nation and author recovering from such traumatic devastation? This paper critically investigates how the problematic of memory invites continuous reflection in a number of issues that emerge in the aftermath of war: the end of a chivalric tradition that opened the way for new literary aesthetics, posttraumatic demands on memory and melancholia, and fantasies of reconstruction in a post-war period of disillusionment. My research problematizes the commonly assumed disjunction between the abstract world of aesthetics and fantasy and the gritty politics of war and power. I argue that Tolkien's literary turn to medievalism and myth provides an alternative to the modernist response to post-war trauma. He revises the chivalric tropes of sacrifice and surrender as a logical ethical and aesthetic response to the brutality of war and the dilemma it raises: how to commemorate the dead, while displacing the logic of war itself. I highlight the importance of negotiating the trauma of war through 'the art of losing,' the narrative by which the lament of loss tempers the valorisation of violence.

Keywords

commemoration – ethics – fantasy – Great War – medievalism – melancholy – memory – mourning – sacrifice – surrender

1 Hugh Brogan, 'Tolkien's Great War,' in *Children and Their Books: A Celebration of the Works of Iona and Peter Opie* (Oxford: Clarendon Press, 1989), 356.

 DOI:10.1163/9789004397576_010

1 The Shadow of the Past

In his "Foreword to the Second Edition,' J.R.R. Tolkien acknowledges the haunting nature of his experiences in the Great War:

> One has indeed personally to come under the shadow of war to feel fully its oppression; but as the years go by it seems now often forgotten that to be caught in youth by 1914 was no less hideous an experience than to be involved in 1939 and the following years. By 1918 all but one of my close friends were dead.[2]

The landscape of *The Lord of the Rings* is shrouded in a menacing darkness about to enslave Middle-earth: the enemy forces are often preceded by sun-blotting mist, and the Dark Lord's chief servants, the Ringwraiths, are creatures of shadow. Yet the shadow is not merely that of individual or even allegorical evil: it also speaks to the psychological devastation of war itself. The language of darkness and despair, then, is in a sense born from the very trauma of contemporary warfare – 'the scars of war and the memory of darkness.'[3]

While Tolkien resisted what he felt was a 'false, though naturally attractive' tendency to apply an author's personal and political experiences upon their literature, he repeatedly returns to the subject of the 'real war' within his own reflections about his work.[4] He delineates the differences between the Great War of Middle-earth and that of the 'real war' in a rebuttal to arguments for an allegorical reading:

> The real war does not resemble the legendary war in its process or its conclusion. If it had inspired or directed the development of the legend, then certainly the Ring would have been seized and used against Sauron; he would not have been annihilated but enslaved, and Barad-dûr would not have been destroyed but occupied. Saruman ... would have found in Mordor the missing links in his own researches into Ring-lore, and before long he would have made a Great Ring of his own with which to challenge the self-styled Ruler of Middle-earth. In that conflict both sides would have held hobbits in hatred and contempt: they would not long have survived even as slaves.[5]

---

2 J.R.R. Tolkien, *The Lord of the Rings*, 50th Anniversary Edition (New York: Houghton Mifflin Harcourt, 2012), iBooks edition, 'Foreword to the Second Edition.'
3 Ibid., Book 6, Chapter 5: 'The Steward and the King.'
4 Ibid., 'Foreword to the Second Edition.'
5 Ibid.

Tolkien distances the 'real war' from the 'legendary war' on several significant fronts, the most significant of which is perhaps in their treatment of power: the legendary war resolves in the destruction of the Ring and with it the potential to enslave Middle-earth by any given party, whereas the 'real war' would not only have resulted in the Ring's seizure and use against Sauron, but also the proliferation of Great Rings created by other parties vying for power. (Intriguingly, Tolkien's description of the power dynamics of the 'real war' bears remarkable similarity to those of the Cold War, which was then just beginning to escalate.) The other significant and related divergence is in the treatment of the powerless: the hobbits humorously distinguished by their diminutive size and disproportionate pleasure in meals and pipes, who 'would have been held in hatred and contempt' by 'both sides ... and would not long have survived even as slaves.'[6] Tolkien's insistence upon the many divergences between the war of his writing and that of the world's reveals his desire to distance his 'legendary war' from the 'real war,' but it also reveals his preoccupation with it: the various ethical dilemmas and dynamics of war influence and shade his mythopoeia, which in turn revises the war in both content and form. It simultaneously engages and disengages with the 'real war.' Whatever else it may be, *The Lord of the Rings* is, inescapably if unintentionally, a post-war epic.

Why, then, revisit medieval and newly compromised tropes in the modern era? *The Lord of the Rings* is a puzzling phenomenon, which draws on medieval tropes to respond to a modern world – with just the hint of a vast, primeval landscape in the background of it all. But it is one that resonates with much of the commemorative artwork following the Great War, which often returned to archaic imagery glorifying sacrifice with images of knights, quests, and spiritualized combat.[7] Historian Jay Winter articulates the ethical and aesthetic struggle to negotiate the tension between valorising and lamenting the deceased that every post-war memorial faced:

> These two motifs – war as *both* noble and uplifting *and* tragic and unendurably sad – are present in virtually all post-war war memorials; they differ in the balance struck between them. That balance was never fixed; no enduring formula emerged to express it, though traditional religious images were used repeatedly to do so.[8]

---

6 Ibid.

7 J. M. Winter, *Sites of Memory, Sites of Mourning: The Great War in European Cultural History* (Cambridge: Cambridge University Press, 1995), 85.

8 Ibid.

On the one hand, there was the ethical obligation to remember the 'noble and uplifting' courage and love involved in a soldier laying down his life for his comrades and country; on the other hand, there was the ethical responsibility to recognize and lament the 'tragic and unendurably sad' violence inflicted upon *and* by the soldier. This unfixable 'balance' persisted as a critical component of the ethical conceptualization of loss. The need to make sense of suffering was an integral component for moving beyond it; deaths became comprehensible only through the conviction that they were 'not in vain,' and yet the justification that they were 'worth it' risked not only downplaying the waste of war, but also paradoxically diminishing the sacrifices it required. Instead of understanding this unfixable 'balance' between the noble/uplifting and the tragic/unendurably sad as a spectrum between two polarized endpoints, what if we were to inhabit this balance as a dynamic tension – the ethical dilemma that negotiates not only the entry into, but also the return from war?

The Lord of the Rings struggles, like so many other post-war narratives and memorials, with the ethical and aesthetic dilemma of how to depict violence: the sacrifice of the soldiers who fell in battle, as well as those who felled others in battle. In response to the modernist critique of medieval tropes, this chapter proposes to complicate the terms of surrender and sacrifice as an ethics of survival that negotiates not only the engagement with war, but also the recovery *from* war. It responds to the enduring call of those who have been lost in the war, the deceased soldier and the dislocated veteran. There are, undoubtedly, many facets of chivalry that have evolved since the Middle Ages; I focus my interest on Tolkien's revision of the tropes of surrender and sacrifice for his contemporary mythopoeia. For his epic is not merely the retelling of old tales, but rather their reinvention in the name of a new national myth. His revision of chivalry develops from his scholarship of medieval texts, but it also develops these notions in moving from an ethos of glory and honour to one of necessity and recovery: his myth represents a critical mediation that reworks the devastation of war. Tolkien problematizes chivalry as an ethical dilemma that responds to the crisis of power abuse, restraining its subjects' exercise of power *against* others, even as it enables power to be exercised *on behalf* of others. As an ethical code, Tolkien's chivalry straddles the tension between restraint and action, simultaneously chastened by the recognition of a universal complicity in evil and spurred by the necessity of courage and conviction in confronting violence – both the physical engagement with violence in war and the psychic violence of post-war trauma.

Writing in the wake of the Great War, which world leaders had promised would be 'the war to end all wars,' Tolkien watched their promises fail and continued to write through the Second World War and the collapse of the

British Empire. *The Lord of the Rings* recovers a medieval space in the modern wasteland upon which the chivalric tropes of surrender and sacrifice play themselves out in encounters between the powerful and the powerless, fantastically reshaping the landscape of Britain in the process. His project navigates the shifting, post-conflict planes of morality and nationalism to reveal the complicity of chivalry in violence, even as it attempts to recuperate its necessity and integrity as a form of witness for the traumatized war veteran of the twentieth century. For the concepts of surrender and sacrifice do not, finally, reduce to naïve ideals that justify bloodshed; they engage the difficulty of leaving battle and returning to life after the encounter with death. Tom Shippey, a scholar of medieval literature, observes of Tolkien's epic, '*The Lord of the Rings* can be taken in itself as a myth, in the sense of a work of mediation, reconciling what appear to be incompatibles … escapism and reality, immediate victory and lasting defeat, lasting defeat and ultimate victory.'[9] It inhabits Winter's unfixable 'balance,' straddling the tension that simultaneously mourns and commemorates the sacrifices undertaken in war. Oscillating between 'escapism and reality,' 'immediate victory and lasting defeat,' 'lasting defeat and ultimate victory,' Tolkien's mediation is ultimately a postwar memorial: the attempt to mediate not only the relationship between the medieval and the modern myth, but also the relationship between the living and the dead.

2 The Art of Losing

Medieval chivalry, as reworked into Tolkien's narrative, did not glorify bloodshed in the name of one's own honour and glory. It moves from valour and violence towards an ethics of necessity and integrity. Necessity provides the motive, while integrity provides the method: it is the recognition of one's own corruptibility in power that drives the restraint of power. In Tolkien's scholarship on medieval heroism, he demonstrates a wary recognition of the dangers of chivalry and its complicity in wasteful and wrongful bloodshed. He writes of Beowulf in 'The Homecoming of Beorhtnoth Beorthelm's Son':

> But the king wished for glory, or for a glorious death, and courted disaster. There could be no more pungent criticism in a few words of "chivalry" in one of responsibility than Wiglaf's exclamation: *oft sceall eorl*

9 T. A. Shippey, *J.R.R. Tolkien: Author of the Century* (Boston: Houghton Mifflin, 2001), xxxii.

> *monig anes willan wraec adreogan,* "by one man's will many must woe endure." These words the poet of Maldon might have inscribed at the head of his work.[10]

Tolkien criticizes Beowulf's rash adventure of seeking to slay the dragon as one of vainglorious folly. He declaims against this brand of chivalry for its 'responsibility' for the suffering of many 'by one man's will.' More to the point, one might also recognize that it is not merely 'by one man's will' that Beowulf's men suffer, but 'for one man's name' – the honour and glory of the king. Tolkien's analysis of Beowulf's 'chivalry' acknowledges elements of waste in the hero, and he rejects the desire for honour and glory, in life and after death, as a legitimizing justification for chivalric action. Such an action, he argues, was both wasteful and wrong. Yet the very recognition that rulers may perpetuate unethical bloodshed also requires its due consideration: how does one restrain and prevent unnecessary force?

The Arthurian legends compiled by Malory grapple with precisely this dilemma of power and the relationship between its exercise and restraint. King Arthur instilled in his knights a code of conduct that undergirded their violence with a combination of initiative and restraint in the Pentecostal Oath:

> [T]hen the king stablished all his knights ... and charged them never to do outrageousity nor murder, and always to flee treason; also, by no means to be cruel, but to give mercy unto him that asketh mercy, upon pain of forfeiture of their worship and lordship of King Arthur for evermore; and always to do ladies, damosels, and gentlewomen succour, upon pain of death. Also, that no man take no battles in a wrongful quarrel for no law, nor for no world's goods.[11]

Here, chivalry mediates the relationship between the individual and the act of violence. Intriguingly, though the Pentecostal Oath is laden with the language of violence, the prolific negatives frame the violence not in terms of aggression, but in restraint: 'never to do outrageousity nor murder,' 'by no means to be cruel,' 'take no battles in wrongful quarrel ... nor for no world's goods.' It is the positive mandates that carry with them the threat of

---

10 J.R.R. Tolkien, 'The Homecoming of Beorhtnoth Beorhthelm's Son,' *Tree and Leaf* (London: HarperCollins*Publishers*, 2001), 150.

11 Thomas Malory, *Works*, 2nd Edition (Oxford: Oxford University Press, 1971), 75.

violence: 'to give mercy ... *upon pain of forfeiture of their worship and lordship of King Arthur* ... to do ladies, damosels, and gentlewomen succour, *upon pain of death*.'[12] Certainly, the phrase 'upon pain of death' need not be read as literally violent, yet it tellingly intertwines suffering and discipline in the definition of the knight's chivalric duties. These duties were to actively aid those in need, but also to restrain them from pursuing violence for 'wrongful' or 'worldly' purposes.

Sacrifice represents a critical intervention into the ethics of war, tempering the valorisation of violence with the lament of loss. For sacrifice, in its primary meaning, is a devotional offering; yet its subsidiary meanings articulate the integral element of substitutionary loss:

> the destruction or surrender of something valued or desired for the sake of something having ... a higher or a more pressing claim; the loss entailed by devotion to some other interest; also the thing so devoted or surrendered.[13]

Sacrifice introduced the concept of loss and wedded it to love, the 'higher or ... more pressing claim' that was *saved*. This move celebrated the love *saved* by the loss, rather than the violence itself, which remained a source of grief in the 'destruction or surrender of something valued or desired.' Within medieval manuals of chivalry outlining the ideals of knightly conduct, the language of sacrifice also supplied the theology that linked them to the Christian tradition. Sacrifice referred to the 'knight's freely willed, voluntary decision to *suffer* in the sacrificial work he undert[ook] – for his lord, for Christ, or for his regiment, as well as for his own glory.'[14] The knight's suffering was often linked to that of the Passion: the death of the innocent Christ to save sinful humanity. Within these medieval manuals, chivalry meant

> above all, discipline, which leads to worthiness that is measured by brave deeds freely undertaken, extending to the greatest distinction, the crown of martyrdom and its promise of proximity to Christ.[15]

---

12 Ibid.

13 'sacrifice, n.' OED Online. March 2013. Oxford University Press, viewed 19 March 2013, http://www.oed.com/view/Entry/169571?rskey=YHJApN&result=1&isAdvanced=false.

14 Allen J. Frantzen, *Bloody Good: Chivalry, Sacrifice, and the Great War* (Chicago and London: University of Chicago Press, 2004), 77–78 (italics added).

15 Ibid., 232.

The motif of the cross is close to the heart of chivalry: the warrior sought the 'crown of martyrdom' because it promised 'proximity to Christ.' Thus, in one sense this image of the king grounded violent 'sacrificial work' in love:

> Chivalry did indeed work against demoralization because it asked men to emphasize love (of all kinds) over hatred. But chivalry did not hide men's violence from them. Instead chivalry squarely centered the warrior's identity on his relationship to violence, on the duties of prowess that formed the center of the circle of chivalry, even as chivalry reminded the warrior that sometimes his duty was to be gentle.[16]

Though the chivalric 'sacrificial work' need not be bloody, it often manifested itself as such in the medieval world. Paradoxical as it may seem to emphasize love as the impetus for potentially violent 'sacrificial work,' the narrative of Christ's sacrifice on behalf of the knight contextualized the knight's suffering on behalf of Christ. The 'circle of chivalry' extended the knight's 'duties of prowess' and protection beyond himself to include a network of others. Sacrifice was, in part, the enactment of Christ's declaration: 'Greater love hath no man than this that a man lay down his life for his friends.'[17] Chivalry evolved as an ethical code to restrain the abuse of power in a movement away from the self through the mandates of sacrifice: service and suffering on behalf of others and a greater good. Sacrifice always entailed the surrender of the self in the name of another; yet this very movement away from the self also opened up the possibility that those who partook in chivalric causes surrendered – along with their 'selves' – a sense of responsibility for their actions. If violence could be justified in the name of another, then what was to prevent the perversion of that name throughout the ages?

The link of violent sacrifice to Christianity provides a problematic contradiction to the underlying logic of the Passion, which was, after all, one of surrendering power to subvert its worldly abuse. Indeed, in the Biblical narrative of Jesus's arrest, Jesus rebukes the disciple who seeks to defend his beloved master by drawing his sword and striking one of the aggressors:

> Put up thy sword into his place: for all they that take the sword shall perish with the sword. Thinkest thou that I cannot now pray to my Father, and he shall presently give me more than twelve legions of angels?[18]

16 Ibid., 265.
17 John 15:13.
18 Matt. 16:52–53.

The death of Christ, though sacrificial, was not the execution but rather the *surrender* of violence: the chilling rebuke and prophesy of perishing against those who would 'take [up] the sword' in the name of love. The Passion itself is an image of 'ultimate victory' in 'lasting defeat' – one in which the sacrifice of the self is tempered by surrender to the other. Yet, as Frantzen notes, 'The death of Abel has been more influential in the history of salvation – and certainly in the history of chivalry – than the death of Christ.'[19] In other words, the innocent blood that cries out from the ground has more often been heard as a cry of revenge than one of reconciliation. In this sense, the history of chivalric violence remains marred not only with the blood of 'enemies,' but also with the betrayal of Christ's sacrifice and surrender.

3 A Difference of Imagination

Ironically, Tolkien negotiates this dilemma of chivalry by foregrounding it: he highlights the corruptibility of his characters through the exercise of power. Part of what renders *The Lord of the Rings* a uniquely contemporary epic despite its medieval ethos is that it is in many senses an anti-epic. It is neither quest, nor conquest: there is no object of power, knowledge, or goodness to be sought after as some holy grail; nor is there a narrative of expansion for power, knowledge, or goodness. There is a ring of power, but it is to be destroyed; there is a lord of power, but his empire must be limited – not replaced. Indeed, these very principles are decided in the first section of the epic during a meeting of the various races resisting the power of the Dark Lord. Boromir, a valiant warrior from Gondor renowned for his feats in battle, proposes that they use the Ring against Sauron:

> Wielding it the Free Lords of the Free may surely defeat the Enemy. … The Men of Gondor are valiant, and they will never submit; but they may be beaten down. Valour needs first strength, and then a weapon. … Take it and go forth to victory!

His perspective is laden with chivalric clichés that define valour as an unwillingness to 'submit' and characterize it by 'first strength, and then a weapon.' Consequently, his view of 'victory' is limited to one of martial besting, and its

19 Frantzen, *Bloody Good.*

method reliant on the seizure – '*Take it!*' – of power. But it is not the vision of the Council. Lord Elrond replies:

> We cannot use the Ruling Ring. That we know too well. It belongs to Sauron and was made by him alone, and is altogether evil. Its strength, Boromir, is too great for anyone to wield at will, save only those who have already a great power of their own. But for them it holds an even deadlier peril. The very desire of it corrupts the heart. Consider Saruman. If any of the Wise should with this Ring overthrow the Lord of Mordor, using his own arts, he would then set himself on Sauron's throne, and yet another Dark Lord would appear. And that is another reason why the Ring should be destroyed: as long as it is in the world it will be a danger even to the Wise. For nothing is evil in the beginning. Even Sauron was not so. I fear to take the Ring to hide it. I will not take the Ring to wield it.[20]

We are given an artefact of power, as exists in so many fantasies and medieval tales, but it is one that must be destroyed. The great power of the ring can only be controlled by those 'who already have a great power of their own,' which initially suggests the familiar paradigm of the duel that pits those with power against each other. However, Boromir's claim that 'valour' relies upon strength and weapons, a notion of honourable combat akin to Beowulf's pursuit of glory, is rejected. It is precisely the powerful for whom the ring holds 'an even deadlier peril,' as power acquires the attributes of addiction: the desire for power 'corrupts the heart.' Even the exercise of power by the Wise 'using [one's] own arts' – that is, the acquisition of dominion through methods and motives which are presumably *not* evil but wise and good – will lead not to the destruction of the Dark Lord, but to the making of a new Dark Lord. Tolkien's work does not explicitly critique Empire, yet it bears a parallel in Sauron, who is characterized by an Eye and a Ring: an Eye that is constantly surveying new lands to conquer, and a Ring that seeks to bind them to his will. The Arthurian notion that might may be used to govern rightly is regarded with a dose of scepticism that there can ever exist a power that is not subject to the methods of exploitation and oppression. The Ring is not to be hidden or wielded, but destroyed: its power must be surrendered.

In his book review of *The Return of the King*, W. H. Auden articulates the primary difference between the good and evil characters not as one of essential

20 Tolkien, *The Lord of the Rings*, Book 2, Chapter 2: 'The Council of Elrond.'

attributes, nor even as one characterized by traditional virtues. Instead, he argues that it is a difference of imagination:

> Evil, that is, has every advantage but one – it is inferior in imagination. Good can imagine the possibility of becoming evil – hence the refusal of Gandalf and Aragorn to use the Ring – but Evil, defiantly chosen, can no longer imagine anything but itself.[21]

The heroes possess the imagination to foresee their own abuse of power, whereas the villains can only imagine themselves. Tolkien moves from an ethics of power-with-responsibility to one that emphasizes power-with-complicity. But as Auden implies, what Tolkien offers in his revision of the quest and conquest narrative is not merely the rejection of power, but also its imaginative subversion: sacrifice with surrender. It is an epic in which not only – or even primarily – the proud and fiery Boromirs are heroes, but also the unassuming and plain-speaking hobbits of necessity. Elrond articulates:

> The road must be trod, but it will be very hard. And neither strength nor wisdom will carry us far upon it. This quest may be attempted by the weak with as much hope as the strong. Yet such is oft the course of deeds that move the wheels of the world: small hands do them because they must, while the eyes of the great are elsewhere.[22]

The 'small hands' moving 'the wheels of the world ... because they must' juxtaposed beside 'the eyes of the great ... elsewhere' echoes the situation of the foot soldier who is a cog in the machinery of the state, whose lofty gaze is removed from the trenches.

4 An Unspeakable Folly

Tolkien subverts the traditional hierarchies and structures of power constrained by an ethic of wartime sacrifice by introducing the term of surrender. Surrender is the unspeakable word in war; the terms of surrender are terms

---

21 W. H. Auden, 'At the End of the Quest, Victory,' *The New York Times*, January 22, 1956, sec. Books, viewed 19 March 2013, http://www.nytimes.com/1956/01/22/books/tolkien-king.html.

22 Tolkien, *The Lord of the Rings*, Book 2, Chapter 2: 'The Council of Elrond.'

of defeat and dishonour. Yet it is the path of necessary wisdom that Gandalf advises to destroy the Ring:

> It is wisdom to recognize necessity, when all other courses have been weighted, though as folly it may appear to those who cling to false hope. Well, let folly be our cloak, a veil before the eyes of the Enemy! For he is very wise, and weighs all things to a nicety in the scales of his malice. But the only measure that he knows is desire, desire for power; and so he judges all hearts. Into his heart the thought will not enter that any will refuse it, that having the Ring we may seek to destroy it.[23]

In an epoch of disorder and destruction, necessity is the only order of the day. But it is not a necessity that is celebrated, but a 'hard road' that 'must be trod.' It is a curious reworking of wisdom in the appearance of folly, and it is stranger yet that it should manifest itself as a rebuke to 'those who cling to false hope.' Given that Gandalf rejects the suggestion that the destruction of the Ring is either the path of despair or folly, the 'false hope' he dismisses is not the possibility of peace, but rather the possibility of peace through power. The Enemy 'weighs all things to a nicety in the scales of his malice,' but his downfall is a myopic vision of his own desire and power that he projects upon everyone else: 'the only measures he knows is desire, *desire for power;* and so he judges all hearts.' He is 'very wise' in his exact calculations, but he is characterized by precisely the lack of imagination – 'into his heart the thought will not enter' – that distinguishes Gandalf as the wiser for envisioning a possibility beyond power, and beyond desire.

The Great War historian Joanna Bourke critiques chivalry because its 'dreams of fellowship gave strength to [soldiers'] violent hands and shrouded the horror of their actions with a mantle of honour.'[24] She argues that it provided a framework in which the 'horror of [warfare]' could not only be 'shrouded,' but also glorified 'with a mantle of honour.' For Tolkien, however, the terms of surrender and sacrifice do not shroud, but rather forefront the corruptibility of power and the ethical dilemma that is chivalry. They centralize and grieve the loss embedded in violence, even as they recognize the necessity of defending *and* dying for certain goods. But what remains a remarkable and relevant reprimand to the valorisation of violence is that this ultimate good 'worth the

---

23 Ibid.

24 Joanna Bourke, *An Intimate History of Killing: Face-To-Face Killing in Twentieth-Century Warfare* (Basic Books, 2000), 359.

sacrifice' is the prevention of the possession of power in the recognition of its corruptibility. Though Tolkien, like Bourke, speaks of a covering – a 'cloak' and a 'veil' – it is not one that masks the devastation of violence with the language of honour: it is the intervention of surrender, the ultimate 'folly' and dishonour in wartime, into the ethics of power and sacrifice.

5 A Long Lost Brother

In *The Lord of the Rings*, one of the noblest characters, Faramir, intervenes in the third volume with history and a sober eye towards war. In a letter to his son, Tolkien puzzled over this new arrival – 'I am sure I did not invent him, I did not even want him, though I like him, but there he came walking into the woods of Ithilien' – who interrupted the action with his history lessons, as well as 'some very sound reflections no doubt on martial glory and true glory.'[25] In the chapters building up to the climactic war of Gondor, Faramir appears for the first time – literally surprising Frodo and Sam from out of the undergrowth, as well as, it seems, their author. We learn that he is the younger brother of the warrior Boromir. Unlike his brother, though, he has no love of battle and a distinctly different vision of glory. He tells Frodo that he would not take the Ring even if his home were in ruins, and he alone could wield it for the good of his country and his glory; he slays neither needlessly nor gladly, and he has no desire for 'such triumphs.'[26] Instead, he contextualizes the war within the framework of necessity – but also, intriguingly, *memory*:

> I would see the White Tree in flower again in the courts of the kings, and the Silver Crown return, and Minas Tirith in peace: Minas Anor again as of old, full of light, high and fair, beautiful as a queen among other queens: not a mistress of many slaves, nay, not even a kind mistress of willing slaves. War must be, while we defend our lives against a destroyer who would devour all; but I do not love the bright sword for its sharpness, nor the arrow for its swiftness, nor the warrior for his glory. I love only that which they defend: the city of the Men of Númenor; and I would have loved her for her memory, her ancientry, her beauty, and her present wisdom.[27]

---

25 Humphrey Carpenter, ed., *The Letters of J.R.R. Tolkien* (London: George Allen & Unwin, 1981), viewed 19 March 2013, http://www.e-reading.by/bookreader.php/139008/Tolkien_-_The_Letters_of_J.R.R.Tolkien.pdf.

26 Tolkien, *The Lord of the Rings*, Book 4, Chapter 5: 'The Window on the West.'

27 Tolkien, *The Lord of the Rings*, Book 4, Chapter 5: 'The Window on the West.'

Faramir grieves the decline of his homeland from the heights of its prosperity, but it is not only the memory of better times he mourns. The 'White Tree' and 'Silver Crown' are metonymies of an era that he himself has not experienced, the Golden Age of Gondor. Since that period, the line of kings has vanished from Gondor for generations; the Stewards, of whom Faramir and Boromir's father is chief, govern the city indefinitely until the return of a royal descendent. Faramir, who is next in line for the Stewardship, longs for the surrender of power to the rightful heir, in a remarkable deviation from his brother Boromir's attitude, who plaints, 'How many hundreds of years needs it to make a steward a king, if the king returns not?'[28] Yet Faramir's depiction of peace is one that distinctly revises the conventional power hierarchies associated with kings; he speaks of queens and beauty, as opposed to kings and strength – a city 'beautiful as a *queen among other queens*: not a mistress of many slaves, nay, *not even a kind mistress of willing slaves*.'[29] Indeed, what is significantly absent from his rhetoric is any mention of brave warriors, bright fortresses, and boisterous brotherhoods; we are presented instead with a vision that is almost akin to an ecosystem of trees, lights, and queens. The significance of this revision of the rule of one (the monarchy) is further revealed in his reference to Minas Anor, as the capitol of Gondor as opposed to Minas Tirith. Faramir longs for the period of relational harmony that the surrender of the Stewardship represents: Minas Anor (the 'Tower of the Sun') is the ancient name for the capital of Gondor. It was only after Minas Ithil (the 'Tower of the Moon'), the companion city of Minas Anor, was seized by Ringwraiths and converted into Minas Morgul (the 'Tower of Sorcery') that Minas Anor became renamed Minas Tirith (the 'Tower of Guard') to respond to the fall of its counterpart as the only remaining defence against Mordor.[30] 'Minas Anor again as of old, full of light, high and fair' is not simply a return to different rulers or even prosperity, but also the restoration of the relationship to Minas Ithil – the destroyed sisterhood and the balance between Sun and Moon, instead of the destructive rivalry and the watchful guard. The war, then, is about more than memory; it is about re-membering history, the knitting together of dismembered limbs to revision 'the White Tree in flower again.'

At first glance, this restorative vision may appear to be one more fantasy that justifies war – another banner that can be borne before one in battle. But if so, it is not one that either shrouds or masks the horror of war, but rather brings it into sharper focus: it is precisely *because* Faramir carries his

28 Ibid.

29 Ibid.

30 Ibid., Appendix A: 'Annals of the Kings and Rulers.'

private grief over Minas Tirith in his heart – the double loss of Minas Anor and Minas Ithil unspoken, but ever shadowing the renamed capitol – that the violence of war becomes all the more grievous. For war represents the antinomy of all that Faramir holds dear in peace: it *is* the 'destroyer who would devour all.' It may be necessary, while there is life, to contend against death – but the struggle for life does not diminish or shroud death; it *heightens* its horror. It is only within this context, then, that love and war can respond to each other in the same paragraph; war may be the negation of love, 'I do not love the bright sword for its sharpness, nor the arrow for its swiftness, nor the warrior for his glory,' but it is also the requirement of love, 'I love only that which they defend ... and I would have loved her for her memory, her ancientry, her beauty, and her present wisdom.'[31] Faramir's intrusion into the narrative, the unanticipated and unknown visitor from Tolkien's subconscious, intervenes into Boromir's bravado; he returns to the scene of war as one from the depths of memory and history, the apparition of a long lost brother with a shock of recognition and an unspoken reminder of another, long lost sister, Minas Ithil.

6 A Medieval Mediation

The intrusion of Faramir into the narrative, like the rupture in the fantastic tapestry of Tolkien's imagination, provides a clue that the fabric of this war-ridden epic may be less the mapping of an entry into or experience of war and more of its return and remembrance. For Faramir's intervention does not, primarily, point to what one 'gets out of war,' but to the dream of *getting out of war*. It is here, in the maze of melancholy, that we find the real relevance of sacrifice and surrender. In his analysis of melancholia, Freud describes the response to bereavement as an open wound, 'drawing to itself cathectic energies ... from all directions, and emptying the ego until it is totally impoverished.'[32] Though bereavement is intuitively concerned with another, the loss of the beloved, it bears a pathological relationship to the 'ego' that has integrated – even consumed – the beloved into its identity. Like war, this wound marshals 'cathectic energies ... from all directions' and sacrifices the ego on the altar of

31 Tolkien, *The Lord of the Rings*, Book 4, Chapter 5: 'The Window on the West.'

32 Sigmund Freud, 'Mourning and Melancholia,' *The Standard Edition of the Complete Psychological Works of Sigmund Freud, Volume XIV (1914–1916): On the History of the Psycho-Analytic Movement, Papers on Metapsychology and Other Works* (Great Britain: Vintage Classics, 2001), 253.

the beloved. War displaces more than lives: it traumatically displaces collective worlds and moral landscapes. The war veteran bears double burdens of grief and guilt over the friends that were killed and those that he killed; in *The Lord of the Rings*, Tolkien's loss may be read into mythic proportions, encompassing not only 'all but one of his closest friends,' but also that of a nation – *Rule, Britannia! Britannia rules the seas!* – and a nostalgically remembered childhood of hobbit-like suburbs that were later industrialized. But in this same psychic realm one also finds these wounds – war itself – reworked in the cathartic counterpart to this draining of 'cathectic energies': the intervention of surrender into the paradigm of sacrifice.

In the aftermath of the climactic battle at Gondor, several of the key characters are struck with a malady described in terms reminiscent of melancholy. The encounter with the Ringwraiths or Nazgûl, creatures of Shadow, leaves psychic scars almost akin to the language of shell shock: '[T]hose who will take a weapon to such an enemy must be sterner than steel, if the very shock shall not destroy them.'[33] When the Shadow of the enemy manifests itself as a malady that falls upon several of the warriors, it takes on a distinctly psychological and spiritual flavour that bears a striking resemblance to depression and despair:

> But now [the doctors'] art and knowledge were baffled; for there were many sick of a malady that would not be healed; and they called it the Black Shadow, for it came from the Nazgûl. And those who were stricken with it fell slowly into an ever deeper dream, and then passed to silence and a deadly cold, and so died. … Still at whiles as the morning wore away [the fallen] would speak, murmuring in their dreams; and the watchers listened to all that they said, hoping perhaps to learn something that would help them to understand their hurts.[34]

Intriguingly, the malady does not simply stem from the physical wounds inflicted by the Ringwraiths, but takes root even if one *inflicts* injury upon the Ringwraiths: it is the encounter with these lords of darkness, not the result of victory or defeat that brings on the malady. This detail highlights the non-physical nature of the malady. The description of its symptom of the ever-deeper dream suggests a detachment from the world akin to depression, and the nightmares of the veterans suffering from post-traumatic stress disorder. But just as the historical doctors were uncertain about what to make of these

33 Tolkien, *The Lord of the Rings*, Book 5, Chapter 8: 'The Houses of Healing.'
34 Ibid.

psychic wounds resulting from a new kind of warfare in the aftermath of the real war, these doctors' 'art and knowledge were baffled' by this malady that left no physical wounds, yet 'would not be healed.' As in both mourning and melancholy, the world becomes bereft of beauty; the stricken fall 'slowly into an ever deeper dream … murmuring in their dreams' that which remains incomprehensible to onlookers – and perhaps even to themselves. We learn that, as in melancholia, the greatest damage is done to the ego: not only does the world become emptied to the stricken, but they also lose the will to live, 'pass[ing] into silence and a deadly cold.' It is difficult to say whether the shadowed more closely resemble those who fell in combat, or those who mourned them. The 'watchers' who listen and wait by their side, 'hoping perhaps to learn something that would help them to understand their hurts,' resemble non-combatants struggling to understand the traumatized soldiers. Yet they also bear similarities with the soldiers themselves, struggling to understand their own experiences.

Sacrifice is a double-edged blade whose two sides of love and loss sharpen each other, neither dulling, both enhancing the bite of the other. Embedded in the depths of suffering is also the poignancy of what it saves, the 'higher claim' that requires the loss. The difficulty of despair stems in part from a kind of traumatic forgetting: the myopic focus upon the edge of suffering, unbalanced by the memory of the saved – and *the memory that has been saved*. The initial stages of the Black Shadow's cure comes in the form of crushing the herb, 'kingsfoil,' and bears psychic dimensions similar to the malady itself. Tolkien describes Aragorn's treatment of the wounded:

> Then taking two leaves, he laid them on his hands and breathed on them, and then he crushed them, and straightway a living freshness filled the room, as if the air itself awoke and tingled, sparkling with joy. … For the fragrance that came to each was like a memory of dewy mornings of unshadowed sun in some land of which the fair world in spring is itself but a fleeting reality.[35]

Ironically, the vital language of 'living freshness' as the 'air itself awoke … sparkling with joy' refers to that of a memory. If memory is that which is remembered in the past, we do not often consider that it could either provide a cure for the present or hope for the future – but that is precisely what the passage suggests. Yet it is a curious memory; like Faramir's memory of Minas Anul, it is a memory beyond past experience: it is a fantasy of a history, of 'unshadowed

35 Tolkien, *The Lord of the Rings.*

sun' and 'dewy mornings.' It is a fantasy that, curiously enough, suggests that the real 'fair world in spring' is 'but a fleeting reality'; it inverts the terms of reality and fantasy, as they have been perverted by the pathological mind. In a sense, then, the reminder of this 'fragrance ... like a memory,' enables the surrender of the lost love object through its substitution with a fantasy. While such a psychic substitution falls short of a full healing – and, indeed, within the narrative the kingsfoil is but the first stage to healing – it is a substitution necessary for survival, which is the precondition to recreating any reality. As Aragorn observes of the wounded Éowyn:

> I have, maybe, the power to heal her body, and to recall her from the dark valley. But to what she will awake: hope, or forgetfulness, or despair, I do not know. And if to despair, then she will die, unless other healing comes which I cannot bring.[36]

The cure enables the regaining of consciousness, intervening into the darkness with the reminder that there is more to sacrifice than suffering, and more to surrender than loss. The 'other healing' will come, eventually, for Éowyn in the substitution of her loss in the transference of her love from the lost object onto another beloved: such is the substitutionary nature of healthy mourning. But this transference is only enabled, first, by the surrender of the beloved. The curative plant, significantly named 'kingsfoil,' participates in Faramir's hope for Gondor and serves as a symbol for the rightful king, whose return heralds the coming peace, but it also reminds the reader that this peace is achieved through sacrifice and surrender: the plant's virtues can only be distilled when it is itself crushed.

7 More than Memory

Faramir's fantasy is in a sense realized. The eventual return of the king, Aragorn, brings first a reminder, and then a manifestation of Gondor's 'memory, her ancientry, her beauty, and her present wisdom.' But he also brings a mediation beyond memory. When he lies down to die, his wife Arwen laments that she must abide 'the loss and the silence' of his death, 'bitter to receive.'[37] He replies with the mysterious words:

36 Ibid.

37 Ibid., Appendix A.

> So it seems. ... But let us not be overthrown at the final test, who of old renounced the Shadow and the Ring. In sorrow we must go, but not in despair. Behold! We are not bound for ever to the circles of the world, and beyond them is more than memory. Farewell![38]

Aragorn leaves his wife with the possibility that though sorrow may be a necessity, despair need not be a natural state of mind. His language parallels that which has been employed throughout the epic to discuss war, as a necessary negotiation. And indeed, the end of war is neither the end nor the limit of loss. Therein lies not only the remaining relevance, but also the lasting applicability of sacrifice and surrender in the engagement of grief. In the reminder of their previous sacrifice, their 'renounce[ment] of the Shadow and the Ring,' remains the potential for a final farewell as the bitter circles of grief become unbound. For Aragorn's words recall, too, the language of mourning and remembrance, by which sorrow need not mean despair, and death need not mean an end. Beyond them is 'more than memory.'

The recognition of sacrifice remains inscribed upon many war memorials, a reminder of the love that does not justify, but lies behind their loss. Whatever Winter may have felt about the inadequacy of 'traditional' responses to war, he acknowledges their power:

> The strength of what may be termed 'traditional' forms in social and cultural life, in art, poetry, and ritual, lay in their power to mediate bereavement. The cutting edge of 'modern memory', its multi-faceted sense of dislocation, paradox, and the ironic, could express anger and despair, and did so in enduring ways; it was melancholic, but it could not heal. Traditional modes of seeing the war, while at times less challenging intellectually or philosophically, provided a way of remembering which enabled the bereaved to live with their losses, and perhaps leave them behind.[39]

Sacrifice became the mediation between the bereaved and the beloved. The 'strength' of the language of sacrifice that drew on medieval modes of expression is in its provision of 'a way of remembering' that does not end, but enables a movement beyond memory. In sacrifice the bereaved may 'live with their losses, and perhaps leave them behind.' Yet though such modes may 'at times'

38 Ibid.
39 Winter, *Sites of Memory, Sites of Mourning*, 15.

be 'less challenging intellectually or philosophically,' they need not always be. Part of chivalry's complexity involved its evolution around the ethical dilemmas of power, and in the aftermath of war its project became no less of an ethical dilemma in the reconciliation – and justification – of anger and grief: in its attempt to validate, if not also valorise, certain kinds of struggle. But the 'strength' of sacrifice is a paradoxical 'power,' because it manifests itself in a critical surrender – the release of the other that frees the self, and the release of power in the recognition of its corruptibility. In revisiting and revising the 'traditional' tropes of chivalry, Tolkien introduced the ethic of surrender into the discipline of sacrifice, opening up a space where that which was unspeakable in war may respond to the unspeakability of war. For *The Lord of the Rings* does provide multi-faceted expressions of 'anger and despair' in 'enduring ways,' and melancholic wounds that do not heal; the difference of this medieval memory is that it also responds to their lasting defeat in a proposal of a different kind of memory, the potential of a fantasy that is ultimately more than memory: the mediation of bereavement.

Those who recite the modern adage, 'Chivalry is dead,' may speak truer than they know. After all, it is only the dead that can truly haunt the living, and loss that fills the mind of the melancholic. In reflecting on the memorials of soldiers from the Great War that drew from medieval imagery, Frantzen writes:

> The proper response to voices from the grave is not sleep but thought and action. But first we must hear them. We think of chivalry as behind us, in the past, merely a backdrop. ... We might think of chivalry instead as a voice calling out from under us.[40]

The medieval voice from the past that calls the soldier into sacrifice is the same voice that calls the survivor out of despair. If it also represents a compromise of necessity and complicity, it is one that is subject to the judgment of not only the living, but also the dead: *The Lord of the Rings* is by no means a pacifist dream, but it is work that engages and reworks the crises of the real war in the legendary one. As Frantzen warns the complacent living who would distance themselves from the bloodguilt of their soldiers: 'These men sacrifice themselves and insist that their motive is love, leaving hatred of enemies to those who do not have to fight them.'[41]

40 Frantzen, *Bloody Good*, 265.

41 Ibid., 242.

Confronted by the call of chivalry in the catastrophe of loss, Tolkien's reworking of sacrifice and surrender as an ethics of survival moves from a revision of the tropes of glory and honour to those of necessity and complicity in war that is ultimately an ethics of release and recovery in its aftermath. In sacrifice and surrender, we find tropes to negotiate not only the soldier's confrontation with his own death, but also the survivor's confrontation with the deaths of the beloved. Frantzen argues that chivalry remains relevant as a justification for war:

> Chivalry reminds us why there is war ... because ideas and traditions can be worth dying for – and worth killing for. Chivalry explains why such dedication, single-mindedness, love, and even bloody-mindedness are, after all, necessary and good.[42]

Sacrifice forefronts loss beside love, the higher claim of 'ideas and traditions ... worth dying for – and worth killing for.' But in Tolkien's work, there opens up the possibility that chivalry may also serve as a reminder of war with all its elements of waste and wrong and a remembrance that moves beyond it in a mediation between the living and the dead. The blood that calls from underneath us is also the voice from beyond the grave, and it is the call to remember that which is more than memory and the possibility of moving on.

Bibliography

Auden, W. H. 'At the End of the Quest, Victory.' *The New York Times*, January 22, 1956, sec. Books. Viewed 19 March 2013. http://www.nytimes.com/1956/01/22/books/tolkien-king.html.

Bourke, Joanna. *An Intimate History of Killing: Face-To-Face Killing in Twentieth-Century Warfare*. Great Britain: Basic Books, 2000.

Brogan, Hugh. 'Tolkien's Great War.' *Children and Their Books: A Celebration of the Works of Iona and Peter Opie*. Oxford: Clarendon Press, 1989.

Carpenter, Humphrey. *J.R.R. Tolkien: A Biography*. Great Britain: HarperCollins, 2002.

Caruth, Cathy. *Unclaimed Experience: Trauma, Narrative, and History*. Baltimore: Johns Hopkins University Press, 1996.

Frantzen, Allen J. *Bloody Good: Chivalry, Sacrifice, and the Great War*. Chicago and London: University of Chicago Press, 2004.

42 Ibid., 263.

Freud, Sigmund. 'Mourning and Melancholia.' *The Standard Edition of the Complete Psychological Works of Sigmund Freud, Volume XIV (1914–1916): On the History of the Psycho-Analytic Movement, Papers on Metapsychology and Other Works*. Great Britain: Vintage Classics, 2001.

Garth, John. *Tolkien and the Great War: the Threshold of Middle-earth*. London: HarperCollins, 2004.

Malory, Thomas. *Works*. 2nd Edition. Oxford: Oxford University Press, 1971.

Rose, Jacqueline. *States of Fantasy*. The Clarendon lectures in English literature. Oxford: Clarendon Press, 1996.

Roth, Michael S. *Memory, Trauma, and History: Essays on Living with the Past*. New York: Columbia University Press, 2012.

Schwarz, Bill. 'Memory, Temporality, Modernity.' *Memory: Histories, Theories, Debates*, edited by Susannah Radstone and Bill Schwarz, 41–60. 1st ed. New York: Fordham University Press, 2010.

Sherry, Vincent B. *The Great War and the Language of Modernism*. Oxford and New York: Oxford University Press, 2003.

Shippey, T. A. *J.R.R. Tolkien: Author of the Century*. Boston: Houghton Mifflin, 2001.

Shippey, T. A. *The Road to Middle-Earth*. Revised and expanded Edition. London: HarperCollins, 2005.

Tolkien, J.R.R. 'The Homecoming of Beorhtnoth Beorhthelm's Son.' *Tree and Leaf*. London: HarperCollins*Publishers*, 2001.

Tolkien, J.R.R. *The Lord of the Rings*. 50th Anniversary Edition. Houghton Mifflin Harcourt, 2012, iBooks edition.

Winter, J. M. *Sites of Memory, Sites of Mourning: The Great War in European Cultural History*. Cambridge: Cambridge University Press, 1995.

CHAPTER 9

The Present and the Future of the Past: the Lasting Gift of the Indian Partition Trauma

Lyda Eleftheriou

Abstract

The wounds of many communities in different parts of the world remain unhealed as they struggle with how to remember traumatic events as well as to reinvent selves and societies. As individual recollection of past events inevitably becomes forever lost, it is crucial to comprehend the process of transmission of a traumatic past. This research paper originates in a number of fundamental and challenging questions regarding the operation of traumatic memory as far as the partition of 1947 in the region of the Indian subcontinent is concerned. These questions relate to how we can appropriately respond to the suffering of the other, the ways that this suffering is handed down and 'remembered' by future generations as well as to the possibility of transformation of the memory of the atrocious events of the Partition to healing, resistance and an altered view of history and our place in it. The cumulative effects of recent events in South Asia, such as the 2008 Mumbai attacks, which derailed the ongoing India-Pakistan peace talks, as well as the ongoing dispute for Kashmir render these questions even more urgent. The aim of this chapter is to delve into exploring the idea of a transgenerational transmission of trauma analysing Amitav Ghosh's *The Shadow Lines* (1988) in order to emphasise its role in creating a liminal space where generations cross the frontiers of time and the ghosts of the past remind us of our ethical responsibility to the suffering other. For this purpose, it invokes Nicolas Abraham and Maria Torok's theory of the phantom, which highlights the psychic effects of the concealed. The analysis of the novel also uses the lens of Marianne Hirsch's concept of postmemory, a concept used to describe the relationship between the children of survivors of collective trauma and the parental experiences.

Keywords

collective trauma – gaps – ghosts – history – Indian partition – memory – phantom – postmemory – silence – transgenerational haunting

•••

 | DOI:10.1163/9789004397576_011

> It is the children's or descendants' lot to objectify these buried tombs through diverse species of ghosts. What comes back to haunt are the tombs of others.[1]
>
> NICOLAS ABRAHAM, *The Shell and the Kernel*

∴

1 A Past That Refuses to Be Past

The wounds of many communities in different parts of the world remain unhealed as they struggle with how to remember traumatic events as well as to reinvent selves and societies. As individual recollection of past events inevitably becomes forever lost, it is of great importance to comprehend the process of transmission of a traumatic past. This research work originates in a number of fundamental and challenging questions about the operation of traumatic memory in regard to the partition of 1947 in the region of the Indian subcontinent. These questions relate to how we can appropriately respond to the suffering of the other, the ways that this suffering is conveyed, sustained and 'remembered' by dwellers of different times and spaces as well as to the possibility of transformation of the memory of the atrocious events of the Partition to healing, resistance and an altered view of history and our place in it. The cumulative effects of recent events in South Asia, such as the 2007 Samjauta Express bombings, which resulted in the death of sixty-eight civilians, and the 2008 Mumbai attacks, which derailed the ongoing India-Pakistan peace talks, as well as the nuclear developments that continue since the 1950s, and the ongoing dispute for Kashmir render these questions even more urgent.

The aim of this chapter is to delve into exploring the idea of a transgenerational transmission of trauma analysing Amitav Ghosh's second novel, *The Shadow Lines* (1988), in order to emphasise its role in creating a liminal space where generations cross the frontiers of time and the ghosts of the past command that we undertake the ethical responsibility we have to the suffering other. For this purpose, it invokes Nicolas Abraham and Maria Torok's psychoanalytic theory of the phantom, which highlights the psychic

1 Nicolas Abraham and Maria Torok, *The Shell and the Kernel: Renewals of Psychoanalysis*, trans. and ed. Nicholas Rand (Chicago: Chicago University Press, 1994), 172.

effects of concealment and the unspoken. The analysis of the novel also uses the lens of Marianne Hirsch's concept of postmemory, a concept used to describe the relationship of the descendants of survivors of collective trauma to the parental experiences. Although the notions of the phantom and postmemory have been developed in connection to individual psychology and the history of the Holocaust respectively, it is the position of this work that they are nevertheless extremely illuminating in the context of transgenerational legacies of collective trauma of other histories and cultures such as that of the subcontinent. This chapter is also written based on the belief that the lives of the descendants of both the victims and the perpetrators involved in traumatic events are greatly determined by the psychic wounds they inherited, albeit in different ways; the analysis of which is beyond the scope of this chapter.

The Shadow Lines belongs to the genre known as a memory novel as it is in essence a recollection of events from the perspectives of the different characters. It has been characterised by Priya Kumar as a 'testimony of loss and memory,' which is critical to our understanding of the Indian partition as a past that cannot be forsaken and that compels us to recognise the transgenerational nature of the violent history of the Partition, its 'past-in-presentness [...] as a history that is not done with, that refuses to be past' by still unravelling and having ramifications vividly felt today.[2]

The refusal of the 1947 Partition to exist only in the past competes formidably against the 'amnesia' of the official nationalist historiography,[3] in both India and Pakistan, concerning the Partition's history of violence. This 'amnesia' towards the trauma of the Partition is combined with the wish of perpetrators to erase the traces of their crimes as well as with the strong resistance on behalf of the survivors to awaken the painful memories of the horrific events that occurred[4] and their actual 'denial of any violence in [their] midst.'[5] Thus, as it is clearly reflected in the novel, it is through the cultural unconscious that the transmission of the trauma of this violent history takes place, that is, through a psychic system of a collective nature, in

2 Priya Kumar, 'Testimonies of Loss and Memory: Partition and the Haunting of a Nation,' *Interventions: International Journal of Postcolonial Studies* 1.2 (1999): 203.

3 Gyanendra Pandey, 'In Defense of the Fragment: Writing about Hindu-Muslim Riots in India Today,' *Representations* 37 (1992): 33.

4 Urvashi Butalia, *The Other Side of Silence: Voices from the Partition of India* (London: Duke University Press, 2000).

5 Gyanendra Pandey, *Remembering Partition: Violence, Nationalism and History in India* (Cambridge: Cambridge University Press, 2001), 188.

which the personal is inseparable from the collective and the political.[6] As Nicholas Rand suggests,

> The falsification, ignorance or disregard of the past – whether institutionalised by a totalitarian state [...] or practised by parents and grandparents – is the breeding ground of the phantomatic return of shameful secrets on the level of individuals, families, the community, and possibly even entire nations.[7]

The collective dimension of the traumatic experiences that occurred during the Partition is indeed of great importance in comprehending that the shattering of families, communities, villages, and cities that took place was in fact the rupturing of a whole way of being in the world as well as the deep scarring of the collective memory. Ghosh's novel evidently illustrates that individual memory cannot be conceived as separate from cultural and collective memory and that consequently, collective memory is vital in sustaining as well as conveying trauma and loss to the next generations.

Thus, although the novel is not situated during the actual upheaval of 1947, the two are so closely interlaced that the Partition's lingering presence in the narrator's life is indeed felt intensely. It is therefore clear that the experience of the transgenerational phantom and postmemory, in contrast to that of mourning or melancholia, involves facing the trauma and the ghosts inherited from an *other*, instead of dealing with what has been directly experienced. Indeed, as Abraham and Torok, as well as Hirsch, describe, the particular story we encounter in the novel is mobilised by unprocessed and unresolved traumas of loss, devastation, shame and guilt relating to a history wounded by slaughter, rape, torture and arson. These are 'liminal experiences that bring us to the abyss of human abjection,' and which result in 'soul murder and social death.'[8] While the narrator 'recalls' them merely as stories and images, with which he was raised, as Hirsch explains, these are nevertheless 'so powerful, so monumental, as to constitute memories in their own right.'[9] The veiled transmission of his antecedents' traumatic experiences by means of storytelling render these memories 'a deeply internalised but strangely

6 Carl Jung, *The Archetypes and the Collective Unconscious* (London: Routledge, 1991).

7 Nicholas Rand, Editor's Note in Abraham and Torok, *The Shell and the Kernel*, 169.

8 Gabriele Schwab, *Haunting Legacies: Violent Histories and Transgenerational Trauma* (New York: Columbia University Press, 2010), 3.

9 Marianne Hirsch, 'Projected Memory: Holocaust Photographs in Personal and Public Fantasy,' *Acts of Memory: Cultural Recall in the Present*, eds. M. Bal, J. Crewe and L. Spitzer (Hanover: University Press of New England, 1999), 8.

unknown past'[10] that consequently haunts the narrator, deeply affecting his sense of belonging and identity and forcing him to embark on a quest for rediscovering it.

Through storytelling, the past is reinvented by the narrator in an endeavour to bridge the rift between bordering generations and shed light onto his personal world in the present. Delving into the past while simultaneously becoming aware of the fact that it must inevitably be reconstructed, or in Hirsch's words, 'recreated,'[11] is an ethical stance that openly competes against the official version of history the narrator grew up with. However, as the narrator says, it is important that we try to reinvent the past 'because [...] if we [don't] try ourselves, we [will] never be free of other people's inventions,'[12] and perhaps more importantly, the forgotten and marginalised will forever remain silent. Consequently, the stories, as carriers of transgenerational trauma, also become seeds of political transformation bearing the promise of change in the way we understand history and our place in it as well as carrying the hope of a 'future-oriented integration of the past.'[13]

2 Casting the Muzzle Away, Finding a Voice

The historian narrator's fascination with unearthing and retelling the past, in a way that uncovers the holes of the dominant versions of historical truth and creates fissures in the national crypt, is obvious in his study of old newspapers, which he says 'transports one in time as nothing else can.'[14] Nevertheless, he is deeply disappointed with the discovery that the newspapers of 1964 in India reduced the communal violence in Dhaka and ensuing riots in Khulna and Calcutta to a mere bottom page story:

> By the end of January 1964 the riots had faded away from the pages of the newspapers, disappeared from collective imagination of 'responsible opinion,' vanished without leaving a trace in the histories and bookshelves. They had dropped out of memory into the crater of a volcano of silence.[15]

10 Eva Hoffman, *After such Knowledge: Memory, History, and the Legacy of the Holocaust* (New York: PublicAffairs, 2004), 6.

11 Marianne Hirsch, 'Past Lives: Postmemories in Exile,' *Poetics Today* 17.4 (1996): 662.

12 Amitav Ghosh, *The Shadow Lines* (Delhi: Ravi Dayal, 1988), 39.

13 Schwab, *Haunting Legacies*, 13.

14 Ghosh, *Shadow Lines*, 279.

15 Ibid., 283.

He tells us that the shroud of silence covering the events of communal violence he experienced in his childhood is: 'So complete [...] that it took [him] fifteen years to discover that there was a connection between [his] nightmare bus ride back to school and the events that befell Tridib and the others in Dhaka.'[16] Silence in this case does not entail the absence of any factual knowledge or positivist account of what occurred, but reveals the absence of any substantial personal or collective psychical processing and therefore the operation of what can be described as a muzzle that prevents this knowledge from acquiring a voice. Since 'Memory is a wounded memory, and the wound seems impossible to heal, to be integrated into history,'[17] it becomes muzzled, shared by everyone but unarticulated.

Referring to his struggle to excavate these events and 'listen' to the silences he says:

> Every word I write about those events of 1964 is the product of a struggle with silence. It is a struggle I am destined to lose – have already lost – for even after all those years I do not know where within me, in which corner of my world, this silence lies. All I know of it is what it is not. It is not, for example, the silence of an imperfect memory. Nor is it a silence enforced by a ruthless state- nothing like that: no barbed wire, no check-points to tell me where its boundaries lie. I know nothing of this silence except that it lies outside the reach of my intelligence, beyond words- that is why this silence must win, must inevitably defeat me, because it is not a presence at all; it is simply a gap, a hole, an emptiness in which there are no words.[18]

His description of this silence as a 'gap,' a 'hole,' 'an emptiness,' which is 'beyond words,' 'outside the reach of [his] intelligence,' vividly echoes Abraham and Torok's position that: 'What haunts are not the dead, but the gaps left within us by the secrets of others,'[19] and therefore reminds us of the phantom, described as lying entombed inside its carrier, hibernating in an intra-psychic 'crypt,' cloaked with secrecy and silence. It is elusive, 'beyond words,' because as the narrator explains:

> The enemy of silence is speech, but there can be no speech without words and there can be no words without meanings – so it follows, inexorably,

16 Ibid., 268.

17 Francoise Vergès, *Monsters and Revolutions: Colonial Family Romance and Mètissage* (Durham, NC: Duke University Press, 1999), 14.

18 Ghosh, *Shadow Lines*, 267.

19 Abraham and Torok, *The Shell and the Kernel*, 171.

> in the manner of syllogisms, that when we try to speak of events of which we do not know the meaning, we must lose ourselves in the silence that lies in the gap between words and the world.[20]

Ghosh thus expresses his reservations and suspicions in regards to the capacity of language to signify the silence that lies within. This is also revealed when the narrator reflects on the state of love and the metaphors used to express this feeling through language:

> And yet between the state and its metaphors there is no more connection than there is between a word, such as mat, and the thing itself: they are utterly indifferent to each other, so that we may heap the metaphors – the diamonds, the suicides, the miles, the suffering – till the end of our abilities, and yet find no trace at all of the state itself.[21]

However, his distrust in words, in language and its power to faithfully correspond to either the external reality or to the hollowness that is hiding deep within, does not deter Ghosh from still believing in the representability of traumatic experience, even if it involves a complete lack of emotional engagement, and in the powerful and empowering qualities of narration in engendering the process of healing and recovery. Nevertheless, since haunting is the symptom of a trauma whose cause 'we do not know the meaning,' and which is 'yet to be determined,'[22] its representation cannot be endeavoured through conventional temporal progression. As Abraham and Torok state, the phantom refuses to die and buried alive, it disrupts the progression of time by attacking language from within and resisting any attempt at being incorporated into one distinct linear narrative.[23] Thus, instead of using conventional linear narrative, Ghosh relentlessly moves amongst shifting times and borders while the narrator weaves an intricate web of political events, from the time of World War II, the partition of Bengal and the late twentieth century, which infiltrate the personal lives of the characters. The narrator's story thus becomes a palimpsest of multiple stories of his grandmother Thamma and her sister Mayadebi, of family friend in London, May Price, his cousins Ila and Robi and of his uncle Tridib. These layers of stories and myriad of voices in effect bend the axis of time, which seems to flow in a cycle forming a spiral maze. They compel the narrator to trace his footsteps

20 Ghosh, *Shadow Lines*, 267.

21 Ibid., 96.

22 Abraham and Torok, *The Shell and the Kernel*, 173.

23 Abraham and Torok, *The Shell and the Kernel*, 175.

back to and from the lacuna in the centre, that is the void created by the traumatic events of the Partition as well as by Tridib's murder in 1964 and the mystery surrounding it. Each individual story, each spiral of the maze, is complex, with many twists and turns, for the maze does not share its secrets easily. On the contrary, it keeps the secret passageways to the crypt well hidden and dark and merely 'stages the verbal stirrings'[24] of the secrets and burdens of the past allowing only a glimpse at them through the relieving and healing act of narration.[25]

Nevertheless, as silence can never be absolute, in its disturbed temporality the particular style of narration in *The Shadow Lines* becomes a sign of the deeply unresolved nature of the historical past of the story. This is fundamental in understanding that the traumatic events of the Partition did not merely take place in time, but have rather shaped the actual experience of time. In other words, as these events remain undigested, never becoming psychically assimilated, they only come into being 'belatedly'[26] and obtain meaning only in connection to another time. Marianne Hirsch argues that this may in fact be predestined as:

> Perhaps it is only in subsequent generations that trauma can be witnessed and worked through, by those who were not there to live it but who received its effects, belatedly, through the narratives, actions and symptoms of the previous generation.[27]

However, as Anne Whitehead points out, if history is characterised by constantly delayed entry into experience, it is then crucial to seriously reconsider the way we view and relate to the past.[28] As the novel reveals, history cannot be considered as fixed objective knowledge, but must be reconceived as an elusive and obscure fluid entity that bleeds into the present and affects not only our sense of selfhood, but also our perception of the world. As Whitehead argues, such a concept of history changes the relation between language and the world, so that from a reflective mode, that aims at self-awareness and

24 Nicolas Abraham and Nicholas Rand, 'Notes on the Phantom,' *Critical Inquiry* 13.22 (1987): 289.

25 Ibid.

26 Cathy Caruth, *Unclaimed Experience: Trauma, Narrative and History* (Baltimore: Johns Hopkins University Press, 1996).

27 Marianne Hirsch, 'Surviving Image: Holocaust Photographs and the Work of Postmemory,' *The Yale Journal of Criticism* 14.1 (2001): 12.

28 Anne Whitehead, *Trauma Fiction* (United Kingdom: Edinburgh University Press, 2004), 13.

self-discovery, the text becomes a performative act, which actively participates in the attempt to perceive and understand the world around us.

Thus, the narrator's movement amongst different times and spaces is more than a mere reflection of the necessity to find an appropriate language to bear testimony to the Partition trauma. It also shows that 'the past is concurrent with the present,'[29] since it inhabits as well as interrupts and moulds it. The lines demarcating past and present generations are therefore reduced in Ghosh's narrative to 'shadow lines' that are too faint and permeable to separate people or generations who share the same history and memories. The narrator is thus led to the 'strangest journey: a voyage into a land outside space, an expanse without distances; a land of looking-glass events.'[30] However, 'the looking glass border' does not reflect distance but rather proximity, the self as 'the inverted image of the other,'[31] the past in the present and the here in the there.

3 Floating between Worlds, Crossing Boundaries

As the narrative unfolds the narrator gradually recognises each of the other characters as his mirror image, a fact that reveals that the self has to be defined not in contrast to the other, but in the way the self and the other relate and connect. The mirror image also reveals that the meaning of difference itself is unreliable and thus interrogates nationalist ideologies that produce the drawing of dividing lines and the erection of barbed wires. This notion is clearly reflected in the narrator's realisation that these divisions, real or imagined, do not necessarily separate people whose identities are different: 'I, in Calcutta, only had to look in the mirror to be in Dhaka; a moment where each city was the inverted image of the other.'[32] The realisation of the irony of borders and of the horror caused by them is more clearly evident in the fact that Tridib is killed on the border, a tragic death, the haunting of which underlies the whole novel, lurking behind the events that occur in the narrator's life.

However, in addition to the obscurity and fictional quality of time and spatial borders, the image of shadow lines also pervades the spheres of imagination and memory in narrating historical truths.[33] Thus, the ghosts of Partition, which

29 Ghosh, *Shadow Lines*, 31.

30 Ibid., 219.

31 Ibid., 286.

32 Ibid., 233.

33 Nadia Butt, 'Inventing or Recalling the Contact Zones? Transcultural Spaces in Amitav Ghosh's *The Shadow Lines*,' *Postcolonial Text* 4.3 (2008): 2.

possess and overwhelm the narrator's entire being, are simultaneously 'ghosts of memory and imagination.'[34] In fact, Hirsch informs us that even memory itself emerges out of an unremitting diffusion between fact and fiction.[35] As a result, the narrator seems to be suspended between the realms of reality and imagination, seeking to comprehend the traumatic memory of Partition in the conjunction between the two worlds, listening carefully to what is suggested by whispers, shadows, gaps and silences. Consequently, real places and events in his memory appear to be as much imaginary as real. This is most vividly manifested in the narrator's description of the room in London where Tridib found shelter from the bombings of the Second World War:

> Slowly, as I looked around me, those scattered objects seemed to lose their definition in the harsh, flat light of the naked bulb; one of their dimensions seemed to dissolve [...] Those empty corners filled up with remembered forms, with the ghosts who had been handed down to me by time: the ghost of the nine-year-old Tridib, sitting on a camp bed [...] the ghost of Snipe in that far corner, [...] the ghost of the eight-year-old Ila, sitting with me under the vast table in Raibajar. They were all around me, we were together at last, not ghosts at all: the ghostliness was merely the absence of time and distance – for that is all that a ghost is, a presence displaced in time.[36]

The ghosts 'handed down' to him 'by time' haunt the room and fill its every corner just like they overshadow his entire existence. Mediated memories become one with unmediated ones so that in the end he cannot distinguish between them. As such, his world transforms into a place in-between where time and spatial boundaries are crossed and generations meet. He himself becomes a place filled with voices emerging not only from the hidden and invisible history of 1947 but also from that of the Second World War and other periods of time.

The narrator therefore allows the boundaries of the 'self' to become porous and receive a multiplicity of others from several generations and geographical spaces. In Abraham and Torok's terms, his identity becomes the shell around a kernel of an 'other' inhabiting an intrapsychic tomb from the beginning. The result is not an identity that is unified and singular, but an 'I' that

34 Ibid., 6.

35 Ofelia Ferrán, *Working through Memory: Writing and Remembrance in Contemporary Spanish Narrative* (Cranbury: Bucknell University Press, 2007), 269.

36 Ghosh, *Shadow Lines*, 222.

is a 'ventriloquist,'[37] through whom a multiplicity of voices that surpassed all boundaries is longing to be heard. In effect, he remains without a name until the end, feeling exiled from the space of his own identity, a condition that is 'characteristic of postmemory,'[38] as well as crucial in becoming the host of the trauma of the other.

However, the narrator says that inescapably, he must be defeated by this trauma: 'I am destined to lose – have already lost,' 'the silence must win, must inevitably defeat me.' This reveals the fact that trauma can never be healed in the sense of a return to the state existing prior to the infliction of the wound. However, it can be worked through when revisited in the process of being 'translated' through storytelling and creative writing. This process of re-engaging with trauma, of mourning, is symbolised in the story by the narrator's gradual but unrelenting removal of the cobwebs covering Tridib's death. His 'memory' of what happened is of course perforated and fragmentary as his efforts focus on piecing together and understanding a history he never experienced by using whatever information he could collect from the stories told as well as from the silences, gaps, sorrow and rage passed down to him by those who experienced the events first hand. Persistently exploring the events that occurred and in the end facing the death of Tridib, however, means coming to the crucial realisation that something has been lost, an acknowledgement which is essential in order to deal with the injuries and gaps created, with the ghosts of the past. In the last page of the novel, realising that Tridib's death was actually a sacrifice that cannot be fully understood, 'for any real sacrifice is a mystery,' he finally feels 'glad' and 'grateful' for 'the glimpse [...] of a final redemptive mystery.'[39]

4 Flowing from the Past through the Present into the Future

Ghosh warns us that exorcising the ghosts of the past means to be relentlessly haunted by them, that the dead cannot be pacified by erasing them from our memories or closing our eyes to their existence. It is only by facing them that we may eventually be led to the very important realisation, which is that individuals and communities across spatial and temporal borders 'are implicated in each other's traumas.'[40] In this way, the formation of new legions against

37 Abraham and Torok, *The Shell and the Kernel*, 173.

38 Hirsch, *Past Lives*, 1996, 421.

39 Ghosh, *Shadow Lines*, 308.

40 Caruth, *Unclaimed Experience*, 24.

horror and violence through sharing and witnessing each other's pain becomes feasible. In Caruth's words, 'In a catastrophic age […] trauma itself may provide the very link between cultures'[41] and hence lead to the imaginative invention of a shared history. The novel is thus an act of summoning the ghosts of the Indian Partition so that we can better recognise our 'entanglements in each other's histories,'[42] so that we can ultimately imagine belonging to communities that do not negate each other.

However, in using the words 'shared history' and 'collective' as well as referring to trauma as having the capacity to create bridges and promote closeness amongst cultures, the fact that the nature of trauma is not universal, but always located in a specific temporal and spatial context, has to be pointed out as well as emphasised. It would, of course, be a mistake to claim that survivors of trauma, or their descendants, in different parts of the world, such as India, Cyprus, Rwanda, and Palestine, do not have many characteristics in common with each other. However, in order to fully grasp the effect of trauma upon a particular community, appreciation and serious consideration of its particular historical, social and cultural dimensions is essential. Unquestionably, this is also a necessity in regards to postcolonial attempts at responding appropriately to and understanding historical trauma and memory.

There is indeed an urgent need for both India and Pakistan to facilitate the development of a culture of memory that includes the bringing of denied pain, secret stories, and intolerable suffering of the traumatic events of the Partition to light. This must involve communal support and the creation of a theoretical framework that can address not only individual but also collective historical trauma. For this purpose, there is a need for a turn towards narratives that consider the political, the psychological, and the social together; narratives that aim at a transformation of the traumatic experience in such a way that emphasis is placed on resilience and survival instead of victimhood and melancholia.

The Shadow Lines, published only four years after the assassination of Prime minister Indira Gandhi and the ensuing sectarian violence that took place in New Delhi, can indeed be seen as belonging together with the narratives that successfully interrogate the way in which differences in South Asia are currently polarised for the purpose of achieving the illusions of unity within each of the two states of India and Pakistan propagated by nationalism. The novel, however, also emphasises that the process of fulfilling our ethical responsibility to the

---

41 Ibid., 11.

42 Shu-li Chang, 'Daughterly Haunting and Historical Traumas: Toni Morrison's *Beloved* and Jamaica Kincaid's *The Autobiography of My Mother*,' *Concretic: Literary and Cultural Studies* 30.2 (2004): 113.

suffering other must focus not only on ways of listening to previously silenced stories, but also on how recovered memory is transmitted from one generation to the next. In this light, Ghosh emphasises the crucial role of literature and the reader who, like the narrator, becomes a secondary witness who receives the narrator's stories throughout the text. The reader thus also becomes haunted in the novel, a feeling that reaches its climax when the haunting quality of the last scene of the novel, in which we have the revelation of how Tridib was murdered, is immediately transferred to the reader.

This transference is achieved as the impact of the revelation of Tridib's death on the narrator's own psychic life is largely withheld. The revelation takes place in the words of May Price, in only three simple lines at the end of the novel: 'When I got there I saw three bodies. They were all dead. They'd cut Kalil's stomach open. The old man's head had been hacked off. And they'd cut Tridib's throat from ear to ear.'[43] These simple words are the product of a seventeen-year-old painful struggle for the narrator, who takes the reader along in participating in the process of 'working through postmemory'[44] having to also invent the story while reading it in order to become free of the inventions of others. The process that Abraham describes as 'placing the effects of the phantom in the social realm,'[45] thus surpasses the textual borders of the novel and in effect includes the reader.

Indeed, the realisation of the importance of addressing the question of how traumatic memory is transmitted is emphasised throughout the novel as the only way for the Indian subcontinent to be able to develop collective practices for working through its violent history. This is certainly a necessary step towards breaking the cycle of the transgenerational transmission of trauma, which renders succeeding generations prone to the repetition of the same historical mistakes and the same violence. The author thus makes an appeal for understanding trauma by listening to 'what can be heard and understood in the voice that speaks through it,'[46] for dealing with psychic deformities such as individual or collective crypts by developing collective practices of mourning that allow feelings suppressed into the cultural unconscious to be processed collectively.

The awareness of the necessity to do so in order to come to terms with the past as well as understand the present and move on to the future, has indeed led numerous authors and artists in recent decades in South Asia to engage

---

43 Ghosh, *Shadow Lines*, 251.

44 Ferran, *Working through Postmemory*, 245.

45 Abraham and Torok, *The Shell and the Kernel*, 176.

46 Caruth, *Unclaimed Experience*, 45.

creatively with the lingering traumatic past they have inherited. The growing number of testimony projects, oral history archives, films, and novels that focus on the Partition all highlight the need for aesthetic and institutional structures that are able to fill the gaps found in historical archives. Nevertheless, the current reality in South Asia testifies to the fact that frictions produced by conflicting interests and desires inevitably spread over to the cultural domain resulting in the politicisation of identities and an escalating conflict dynamic in which the other is regarded as threatening and problematic. The outcome is of course a national inability to mourn as well as an atmosphere of doubt, distrust, and aggression, in which efforts to dominate and suppress adversaries displace initiatives to join forces in search for mutual political accommodation.

Recent occurrences such as the extremely formidable reaction of many locals, in 2012, to the possibility of renaming a busy traffic circle in Lahore after Bhagat Singh, a non-Muslim local hero, as well as the well-known Ayodhya Debate, which resulted in the demolition of the Babri Mosque as well as the death of two thousand people in subsequent riots in India, in 1992, all point to the fact that social memory is fundamental to the creation of social meaning and that representations of the past shape the imagining of a community. What is at risk of becoming lost in the struggle to define the past is thus great, a fact that renders social memory an important site of political dispute and opposition. It is thus clear that the power of the two nation-states of India and Pakistan is crucially constituted by representations of a national past, one that excludes the violence of the Indian Partition, the memories of survivors, the horror and brutality of the time as well as the often idealised pre-partition era when Muslims, Hindus and Sikhs lived together in an atmosphere that was in general harmonious and peaceful. This exclusion of course constitutes part of the effort through which the past, the history of the nation, is moulded in such a way so as to embody nationalist values entirely. The past that cannot be accepted and tolerated, that is judged to be inappropriate for public consumption, has been expelled from national history and the fact that the creation of a Partition Museum has never materialised, despite several initiatives in both states, is also a reflection of that effort made by each state.

However, the fact that there are voices that dare to challenge official truth and struggle against the efforts that try to marginalise and silence them, as well as the existence of those who insist on revisiting the trauma of Partition, reveal the truth about the relationship between popular and dominant memory, which cannot be fixed. On the contrary, it remains fluid, constantly negotiated. As history constitutes the premises of an incessant war between India and Pakistan, there is always potential for challenging dominant versions of truth, even where the influence of official ideology is compelling. Standing between the borders of now and the future, *The Shadow Lines* thus urges its readers to begin to move forward with a sense of collective responsibility to the silenced other, including not only those with whom they share the same history and culture, but also the inhabitants of all times and places whose suffering originates in either tangible or imagined divisions.

Bibliography

Anderson, Benedict. *Imagined Communities: Reflections on the Origin and Spread of Nationalism*. London: Verso, 1983.

Abraham, Nicolas and Maria Torok. *The Shell and the Kernel: Renewals of Psychoanalysis*. Translated and edited by Nicholas Rand. Chicago: Chicago University Press, 1994.

Abraham, Nicolas and Nicholas Rand. 'Notes on the Phantom: A Complement to Freud's Metapsychology.' *Critical Inquiry*, 13.2 (1987): 287–292.

Butalia, Urvashi. *The Other Side of Silence: Voices from the Partition of India*. London: Duke University Press, 2000.

Butt, Nadia. 'Inventing or Recalling the Contact Zones? Transcultural Spaces in Amitav Ghosh's *The Shadow Lines*.' *Postcolonial Text* 4.3 (2008): 1–16.

Caruth, Cathy. *Unclaimed Experience: Trauma, Narrative and History*. Baltimore: Johns Hopkins University Press, 1996.

Chang, Shu-li. 'Daughterly Haunting and Historical Traumas: Toni Morrison's *Beloved* and Jamaica Kincaid's *The Autobiography of My Mother*.' *Concentric: Literary and Cultural Studies* 30.2 (2004): 105–27.

Felman, Shoahana and Dori Laub. *Testimony: Crises of Witnessing in Literature, Psychoanalysis, and History*. New York: Routledge, 1991.

Ferrán, Ofelia. *Working through Memory: Writing and Remembrance in Contemporary Spanish Narrative*. Cranbury: Bucknell University Press, 2007.

Ghosh, Amitav. *The Shadow Lines*. Delhi: Ravi Dayal, 1988.

Hirsch, Marianne. 'The Generation of Postmemory.' *Poetics Today* 29.1 (2008): 103–128.

Hirsch, Marianne. 'Projected Memory: Holocaust Photographs in Personal and Public Fantasy.' *Acts of Memory: Cultural Recall in the Present*, edited by M. Bal, J. Crewe, and L. Spitzer, 3–23. Hanover, NH: University Press of New England, 1999.

Hirsch, Marianne. 'Past Lives: Postmemories in Exile.' *Poetics Today* 17.4 (1996): 659–686.

Hirsch, Marianne. 'Surviving Image: Holocaust Photographs and the Work of Postmemory.' *The Yale Journal of Criticism* 14.1 (2001): 5–37.

Hoffman, Eva. *After such Knowledge: Memory, History, and the Legacy of the Holocaust*. New York: PublicAffairs, 2004.

Jung, Carl. *The Archetypes and the Collective Unconscious*. London: PublicAffairs, 1996.

Kaplan, Ann E. *Trauma Culture: The Politics of Terror and Loss in Media and Literature*. New Brunswick, NJ: Rutgers University Press, 2005.

Kumar, Priya. 'Testimonies of Loss and Memory: Partition and the Haunting of a Nation.' *Interventions: International Journal of Postcolonial Studies* 1.2 (1999): 201–215.

Leys, Ruth. *Trauma: A Genealogy*. Chicago and London: The University of Chicago Press, 2000.

Pandey, Gyanendra. 'In Defense of the Fragment: Writing about Hindu-Muslim Riots in India Today.' *Representations* 37 (1992): 27–55.

Pandey, Gyanendra. *Remembering Partition: Violence, Nationalism and History in India*. Cambridge and New York: Cambridge University Press, 2001.

Rand, Nicholas T. Introduction to *The Shell and the Kernel*, by Nicholas Abraham and Maria Torok, 1–22. Chicago: Chicago University Press, 1994.

Sen, Asha. 'Crossing Boundaries in Amitav Ghosh's *The Shadow Lines*.' *Journal of Commonwealth and Postcolonial Studies* 5.1 (1997): 46–58.

Schwab, Gabriele. *Haunting Legacies: Violent Histories and Transgenerational Trauma*. New York: Columbia University Press, 2010.

Vergès, Francoise. *Monsters and Revolutions: Colonial Family Romance and Mètissage*. Durham, NC: Duke University Press, 1999.

Whitehead, Anne. *Trauma Fiction*. United Kingdom: Edinburgh University Press, 2004.

CHAPTER 10

Finding the Way Home: an Interdisciplinary Perspective on Trauma and Trauma Resolution Practices

Stefanie Marie Margarete Dinkelbach

Abstract

This chapter proposes a perspective that focuses on the loss of a sense of connection as an effect of trauma, thereby facilitating a comparison between individual psychology and the micro – and macro-social levels. Studies from a variety of disciplines including neurobiology, psychology, psychotherapy, sociology, and history will be combined to show how a sense of interconnectedness on a personal, social, and collective level can become disturbed by trauma or trauma-like experiences. Interconnectedness on a personal level is facilitated through the ability of the brain to fluently adapt to change, which is disrupted by the persistent and out-of-context nature of traumatic memory. In the group related and societal context it is a sense of social connection and belonging that can become disturbed by experiences of grief, shame, and humiliation as well as by social alienation and dislocation. The link between such disruptions of connectivity and violence shows the need for processes that facilitate a reconnection and a variety of approaches will be discussed ranging from therapy methods to group based and societal interventions including representational processes. Drama productions that use the element of absurdity and 'Butoh', a contemporary Japanese dance format, are discussed as examples in this context. Restorative processes that aim to facilitate reconnection through recognition can make a most relevant contribution by turning the disruptive potential of the experience into an opportunity for personal growth and awareness. However, it is argued that a sustainable prevention of retraumatisation can only be achieved through a fundamental change in perspective towards a world-view that is based on a sense of interconnectivity rather than on fear. To revise the fear-based perspective that informs our society and has caused experiences of disconnection that can be traced through European history, Marshall Rosenberg's concept of Nonviolent Communication is proposed as a possible approach.

 | DOI:10.1163/9789004397576_012

Keywords

cultural representation of trauma – memory formation – nonviolent communication – post-traumatic growth – trauma – trauma therapy

1 Introduction

Peter Levine describes trauma as a loss of connection that affects the individual in its relation to itself as well as with its social and natural environment. The healing of trauma must therefore be, according to Levine, a restoration of this lost connection.[1] This perspective that refers to the context of individual psychology will be extended in this chapter to the micro- and macro-social level, where events and experiences can be observed to cause a similar loss of connection in the social environment.

To make this comparison possible, an in-depth enquiry into the traumatisation process is necessary, one that shows on the level of neurobiology a pattern formation that verifies Levine's observation. The pattern in which an initial state of connection becomes disrupted can also be detected in the social context where experiences or events cause a sense of disconnection. The link that can be observed between such experiences of disruption and violence makes the urgent need for restorative processing apparent. A variety of approaches that attempt to facilitate a reconnection both on the level of individual psychology and in the social context will be discussed briefly in this chapter. Ranging from trauma therapy methods to social and societal interventions, the discussion will also include representational processes that are facilitated by cultural productions.

While trauma and trauma-like experiences that cause a disrupted sense of interconnectedness can be reprocessed to facilitate a restoration of the lost sense of connection, it is important to raise awareness of the fact that our Western society is based on a sense of disruption that informs the way in which we relate to ourselves as well as to our natural and social environment. This lost sense of connection in the form of a fear-based perspective in which some are perceived as 'others' can be traced through European history as a legitimising concept that facilitates violence. A revision of this perspective is hereby seen as a precondition to both trauma resolution and violence prevention and as a

1 Peter Levine, 'Nature's Lesson in Healing Trauma,' viewed 26 January 2013, 18, http://trauma-healing.com/somatic-experiencing/reference-healing-trauma-lessons-from-nature.pdf.

move towards a restoration of our sense of interconnectedness that is fundamental as well as sustainable.

2 Methodology

To recognize processes that show a pattern formation that facilitates the comparison between the level of individual psychology and the micro- and macro-social levels, studies from a number of disciplines including neurobiology, psychotherapy, psychology, sociology and history will be referred to. While the interdisciplinary approach that is used here is needed to facilitate the exploration of trauma from a variety of perspectives, it necessitates a certain amount of simplification of areas that are otherwise very complex. The underlying truths or principles that are outlined here should, despite this simplification, still be accurate.

3 The Disruptive Nature of Trauma Memory

To understand how trauma can disrupt a predisposition towards interconnection, it is necessary to look at the processes involved in memory formation.

Eric Kandel explains that what we call memory is facilitated by a connection between brain cells through synapses. Synaptic connections are established in response to sensory stimuli, maintained by proteins if the stimuli persist and pruned when no further stimulation is received as proteins decay naturally. The loss of the synaptic connections causes the loss of the memory of the original stimulation, a process that we call forgetting.[2] This ability to adapt to user demand, which Joseph LeDoux calls 'synaptic plasticity'[3] or plasticity of the brain, enables the individual to respond to his or her present environment and to adjust to its changing conditions whenever necessary. It can thereby be identified as a pre-dispositional state of interconnection that provides the individual with a sense of interrelatedness and an ability of being present in the present moment.

A traumatic experience can disrupt this state of interconnection. According to Kandel, the extreme stimulus of a traumatic event can cause the formation of a prion-like protein (prion standing for 'proteinaceous infectious agent', an infectious protein that can cause degenerative diseases of the

2 Eric Kandel, *In Search of Memory* (New York: Norton & Company Inc., 2006) 275.
3 Joseph LeDoux, *Synaptic Self* (New York: Penguin, 2002), 9.

nervous system). This 'infectious' protein has the ability to perpetuate itself. It can therefore maintain the synaptic connection indefinitely, irrespective to user demand.[4] The memory that is in this way maintained can resurface suddenly and out of context thereby disrupting the ability to adapt and respond. The persistent nature of the trauma memory, therefore, creates a rupture between the individual and his or her environment and its continuously changing circumstances.

While the traumatic memory is persistent, it is also in most cases implicit. It is the difference between a fear-based response under normal circumstances and a response under extreme threat that explains the implicit nature of trauma memory.[5] David Lisak describes how sensory stimuli are, under normal circumstances, processed by an array of neural pathways in which the cortex is included, thereby facilitating conscious decision-making and conscious memory. As this process is time consuming, it is not appropriate in a life-threatening situation where fast reaction is crucial to survival. Stimuli that signal extreme threat therefore bypass the cortex and reach the amygdala directly, an ancient part of the brain that processes emotions and stores implicit memory. In the struggle for survival the amygdala activates the autonomous nervous system, which enables the release of hormones that initiate changes in the body and facilitate a fight, flight or freeze response. This fast and effective process does not allow for the mediation of stimuli and can, according to Robert Scaer, overwhelm the amygdala.[6] It is these extreme stimuli that can cause the formation of prion-like proteins that, being able to perpetuate themselves, maintain a synaptic connection indefinitely. The persistent and implicit memory of the traumatic event that is in this way formed can cause the symptoms of Post-Traumatic Stress Disorder. These symptoms include:

1. Flashback memories as a reactivation of traumatic memory triggered by stimuli that resemble those of the initial trauma-inducing event. The sudden and out-of-context nature of the reoccurrence disrupts the individual's relation to the present.[7]
2. Hysteria as an expression of excessive fear, which is caused by a self-sustaining cyclical reaction that can occur when the amygdala in its over-stimulated state sends signals that mediate arousal to a number of brain

4 Kandel, *In Search of Memory*, 273.

5 David Lisak, 'The Neurobiology of Trauma,' (unpublished article, 2002), 1, viewed 29 August 2009, http://id3464.securedata.net/nowldef/html/njep/dvd/pdf/neurobiology.pdf.

6 Robert Scaer, 'The Neurobiology of Dissociation and Chronic Disease,' *Applied Psychophysiology and Biofeedback*, 26.1 (2001), 75.

7 LeDoux, *Synaptic Self*, 257.

centres which, once activated, return the signal thereby further reactivating the amygdala.[8]

3. Compulsive trauma re-enactment, as the result of an addictive behaviour that a victim of trauma develops to the anaesthetising effect of a hormone that is released during trauma response. Through the addiction the individual is drawn towards a re-enactment of the initial trauma-inducing event in a way that is compulsive.[9]
4. Dissociative disorders, as personality disorders that are caused by a withdrawal response to an experience of extreme threat. While the withdrawal response, which is related to the freeze reaction, facilitates survival under otherwise overwhelming circumstances, it can leave a dissociative behaviour pattern.[10]

A link between post-traumatic symptoms and violence is particularly apparent in the post-traumatic symptoms related to dissociation and compulsive re-enactment. While dissociation facilitates the occurrence of violence through the passive composure that it causes, the connection between compulsive re-enactment and violence is more obvious, and according to Peter Levine, compulsive trauma re-enactment is a major contributor in the escalation and perpetuation of violent behaviour.[11]

The symptoms of PTSD that are listed here represent some of the pathologies of Shock Trauma. Similar but often more varied and pervasive symptoms occur in relation to Developmental- or Complex-Trauma, which can, according to Bessel van der Kolk, be caused by prolonged stress and repeated traumatisation, particularly when experienced in early childhood.[12]

4 Loss of Interconnectivity in the Micro-Social Context

The predisposition towards interconnectivity in the micro-social setting can be identified as an inclination towards social connectedness and interactions that produce a feeling of group solidarity. Randall Collins who focuses on micro-social processes talks about a micro-rhythm that every participant brings into a group interaction. According to Collins, participants tune into each

8 Ibid., 290.

9 Scaer, *Neurobiology of Dissociation and Chronic Disease*, 77.

10 Ibid., 73.

11 Peter Levine, *Healing Trauma* (Boulder Co: Sounds True Inc., 2005), 4.

12 Bessel A. van der Kolk, 'Developmental Trauma Disorder,' *Psychiatric Annals*, 35.5 (2005), 2.

other's micro-rhythms during interaction rituals, which produces a sense of social connectedness and amplifies the amount of emotional energy that every participant brings into the interaction. This amplification results in an increase in emotional energy for each contributor. Collins highlights the importance of emotional energy in stimulating, through the action of neurotransmitters and the flow of hormones in the endocrine system, a feeling of happiness as well as active behaviour.[13] Access to interaction rituals that enable emotional energy gain through this form of 'rhythmic entrainment'[14] can thereby be seen as necessary on a biological level and according to Collins a common desire towards a sense of social connectedness can be observed in combat as soldiers generally show great difficulties in overcoming this tendency.

A sense of a loss of social connection can be experienced through the emotions of grief, shame and humiliation. According to Helen Lewis, shame, as an experience of loss of social bonds, signifies in the case of an infant a threat to survival. Lewis found that psychotherapy clients would express hostility after an experience of unacknowledged shame.[15] For Thomas Scheff a loss of a sense of social connection through experiences of grief, shame and humiliation can be the source for hatred and the hidden component of rage and aggression.[16] Scheff in his inquiry into the emotional/relational causes for violence identifies a pattern of emotional management in which unacknowledged shame and humiliation are significant contributors. This form of emotional management, which Scheff calls 'hypermasculinity', is characterised by a silence/violence pattern and can, due to cultural conditioning be found predominantly in men, while a female equivalent displays obedience, blind loyalty and fearfulness as character traits. According to Scheff, women that adopt the pattern of hyperfemininity are attracted to their male hypermasculine counterparts and the two mutually reinforcing hypergenders contribute towards a social atmosphere that promotes conflict and war.[17]

---

13 Randall Collins, *Interaction Ritual Chains* (Princeton NJ: Princeton UP, 2004), 106–107, 120.

14 Ibid., 120.

15 Helen Lewis, 1971, in Thomas J. A. Scheff, 'Theory of Runaway Nationalism: Love of Country/Hatred of Others,' (unpublished manuscript, 2006), 5, viewed 8 March 2009. http://www.soc.ucsb.edu/faculty/scheff.

16 Scheff, 'Theory of Runaway Nationalism: Love of Country/Hatred of Others,' 6.

17 Thomas J. A. Scheff, 'War and emotion: Hypermasculine Violence as a Social System,' (unpublished manuscript, 2007), 12, viewed 8 March 2009, http://www.soc.ucsb.edu/faculty/scheff.

Evelin Gerda Lindner identifies the dynamics of humiliation as the core agent in conflict that escalates into cycles of violence.[18] Lindner differentiates between humiliation and shame and highlights the element of degradation as a particular characteristic of humiliation which she defines as an 'enforced lowering of a person or a group, a process of subjugation that damages or strips away their pride, honour and dignity'.[19] According to Lindner, depression is often the first reaction to a humiliation experience, followed by the desire to retaliate with aggressive counter-humiliation that can range from sabotage to more overt forms of aggression depending on the resources available to the victims.[20]

The causal link between violence and a sense of lost social connection through unacknowledged experiences of shame, grief and humiliation as shown by Lewis, Scheff and Lindner is further explained by Collins' observations on interaction rituals where domination is achieved. Collins describes how such interaction rituals can emerge out of an encounter between participants who are low but not equally low in emotional energy and whose micro rhythms are misattuned. The participant with the relatively higher amount of emotional energy struggles to establish an authoritative rhythm over the other participant and recuperates the emotional energy that the victim loses in the process of domination.[21] When access to interaction rituals becomes restricted due to a sense of loss of social connection, this form of interaction can become an alternative means of gaining emotional energy.

5 Loss of Interconnectivity in the Macro-Social Context

A pattern in which the disposition towards interconnectivity is lost can also be identified on the macro-social level. In this context it is a sense of group cohesion that can be identified as the state of interconnection that can become disrupted by events that cause social dislocation and alienation. War, revolution, and natural disasters have the potential to have such a disruptive effect on the macro-social scale. Industrialisation and modern capitalism have been perceived by modernist theorists such as Anthony Giddens and Thomas Nairn as developments that

18 Evelin Gerda Lindner, 'Healing the Cycles of Humiliation: How to Attend to Emotional Aspects of "Unsolvable Conflicts" and the Use of "Humiliation Entrepreneurship," *Peace and Conflict*, Journal of Peace Psychology, 8.2 (2002), 125.

19 Ibid., 127.

20 Ibid., 132.

21 Randall Collins, *Violence* (Princeton NJ: Princeton UP, 2008), 135, 189.

caused widespread experiences of social crisis.[22] George Mosse refers to the sudden and extreme nature of the Industrial Revolution in Germany, which gave the population no time to adjust to the fundamental changes that their social reality had been subject to.[23] As the production capacity in Germany increased by 800% between the years 1870 and 1913[24] a number of social groups, especially peasants, craftsmen and members of the lower middle class were, according to Mosse, directly affected by this drastic change and threatened with the loss of both their social status as well as their livelihood. Mosse describes the sense of lost connection that affected German society at the time:

> [S]urrounded by an encroaching industrial society, men and women looked for a deeper meaning in life than the transitory reality of their present condition. The rapid process of European industrialization was indeed bewildering to them, accompanied as it was by the dislocation of the population, by the sudden obsolescence of traditional tools, crafts and institutions and by social maladjustment and upheaval. The demands of an increasingly industrial society, with its new opportunities and restrictions tended to strengthen the individual's feeling of isolation. This isolation, man's alienation from both himself and his society, occupied men as divergent as Tocqueville and Karl Marx.[25]

The climate of social alienation contributed, according to Mosse, towards a sense of uprootedness that made the German population susceptible to ideological distortions. Mosse refers to an ideology of the Volk nature and race that was particular to Germany[26] and later developed into fascism, which was heralded as the antidote to the fragmented nature of society.[27]

6 Restoration of Interconnectivity

A sense of lost connection can be addressed in such a way that a reconnection is fostered and the many methods and approaches that have developed

---

22 Anthony Giddens, *Social Theory and Modern Sociology* (Stanford: Stanford UP, 1987), 34; Thomas Nairn, *The Break-up of Britain* (London: New Left Books, 1977), 97–8.
23 George Mosse, *The Crisis of German Ideology*, (New York: Schoken Books, 1964), 13–14.
24 Peter Pulzer, *Germany 1870–1945* (Oxford: Oxford UP 1997), 16.
25 Mosse, *Crisis of German Ideology*, 13–14.
26 Ibid., 315.
27 Ibid., 313.

to facilitate such a form of reprocessing share the same underlying principle. Whether on the level of individual psychology or in the social and societal context, it is the recognition that the disruption has occurred and the increase in awareness that this recognition causes that enables the restoration process.

In individual psychology, therapy methods have been developed to facilitate a revisiting of the original trauma inducing experience under non-threatening circumstances. The establishment of a sense of emotional and physical safety is therefore a precondition in this process, in which the trauma memory as the element of disruption is identified through cognitive or implicit processes that encourage its release. The most noteworthy methods in relation to this enquiry are:

1. Traumatic Incident Reduction (TIR), a procedure that uses regressive desensitisation to encourage reduction and elimination of the negative effect of traumatic memory. TIR traces the occurrence of post-traumatic symptoms in a patient's life to identify the original trauma-inducing event. The patient is guided to revisit this experience in a one-to-one imaging process that encourages reprocessing through cognition.[28]
2. Somatic Experiencing, a trauma therapy method developed by Levine, that tracks the traumatic experience through its impact on the body by looking at the disregulation of the autonomic nervous system that has been caused by trauma. The therapy establishes the patient's ability to return to a safe and regulated state and then alternates between briefly visiting the disregulated state, through trauma recall, and returning to the regulated state, until the fear inducing memory can be re-experienced as safe.[29] The persistent implicit memory of extreme threat is in this way replaced with a conscious, non-persistent memory that can be released as the autonomic nervous system returns to its ability to self-regulate.
3. Eye Movement Desensitization Reprocessing (EMDR) employs a variety of aspects of traditional psychological therapy methods to encourage a revisiting of the original trauma inducing experience. Alternating left-right attention or regular sound beats are used to reprocess the stored trauma memory during recall by turning on the brain's rapid eye movement sleep system, which facilitates the integration of traumatic memory into semantic networks.[30]

---

28 Robert H. Moore, 'Background and Theory of Traumatic Incident Reduction,' in V. R. Volkmann, ed. *Traumatic Incident Reduction: Research and results* (Michigan: Loving Healing Press, 2005), 14.

29 Levine, 'Nature's Lesson in Healing Trauma.'

30 Uri Bergmann, 'Further thoughts on the Neurobiology of EMDR: The Role of the Cerebellum in Accelerated Information Processing,' *Traumatology* 6 (2000), 175–200.

It is the identification of the disruption that leads to an increased awareness, which facilitates the restoration of the lost connection, not only on the level of psychology, but also in the micro- and macro-social context.

Lindner states that an awareness of the dynamics of humiliation is necessary to confront and break its self-perpetuating cycle. Speaking from personal experience as a victim of humiliation and with a focus on actions that individuals can take to minimise their own contribution in the humiliation/counter-humiliation process, she stresses the need for victims as well as perpetrators to recognise and acknowledge their position in and their contribution to the humiliation/counter-humiliation process. She highlights the importance of the victims' recognition of the role that their own feelings of inferiority and admiration for the otherwise despised superior play in this context. Lindner sees the process of confronting and healing the cycles of humiliation as an interpersonal as well as a societal undertaking.[31]

According to Collins, an increased awareness of the mechanisms of micro-social interaction can prevent a situation in which one becomes caught up in their violent dynamics. He gives a number of practical recommendations in relation to violence prevention which include: an awareness of the dynamics of what Collins calls 'forward panic' in relation to the police force as well as to the military, a knowledge of the street codes in violent districts, an awareness of the dynamics of dominant interaction that can prevent victimisation and a recommendation to make blustering an equal sided ritual that facilitates the letting go of tension rather than allowing it to develop into violent action.[32]

For Scheff it is the acknowledgment of experiences of grief, shame and humiliation that can remedy a situation that holds the potential for violence. This acknowledgement can, according to Scheff, happen on the interpersonal as well as on the macro-social scale through public events that may take the form of collective rituals.[33]

Jeffrey C. Alexander describes a process in which experiences of a lost sense of social connection are publicly acknowledged in a way that encourages collective awareness. In what he refers to as the 'social process of cultural trauma'[34] the traumatic nature of an event must be claimed through a new master narrative. Alexander stresses that this new narrative needs to

31 Lindner, 'Healing the Cycles of Humiliation,' 135.

32 Collins, *Violence*, 464–466.

33 Scheff, 'War and emotion,' 14.

34 Jeffrey C. Alexander, 'Towards a Theory of Cultural Trauma,' in *Cultural Trauma and Collective Identity*, Jeffrey C. Alexander, ed. (California: UP Berkeley, 2004), 10–11.

acknowledge and raise awareness of the nature of the sense of rupture that has occurred, who has been affected by it, how the audience is related to the event and its victims and how this rupture has been caused.[35]

The social process of cultural trauma as described by Alexander, is in many ways comparable to the methods of trauma therapy discussed previously. Rather than recalling the initial trauma inducing experience, it is in this case the event that caused the sense of disruption to the collective that is reinvoked through a new narrative that calls for public recognition and awareness. The acknowledgment by the collective that alienation and dislocation has been experienced, contributes towards a raised awareness that restores the lost sense of collective belonging.

7 Cultural Productions as Contributions to the Resolution Process

As cultural productions have the potential to raise awareness in a collective setting, they can play a key role in the social process of cultural trauma as described by Alexander. A variety of approaches have developed in response to experiences of social cohesive loss that facilitate the establishment of a new narrative in which the collective faces and acknowledges the occurrence of a ruptured interconnectivity. Since collective experiences of crisis often foster the emergence and establishment of narratives that offer divergence and an escape into a realm of imaginary safety, the deconstruction or replacement of such, often conventionalised, narratives becomes a precondition in this process.

Among the different approaches that facilitate the formation of a new narrative, it is the establishment of a counter-narrative that challenges existing conventionalised accounts, that is the most common and accessible. This approach is used in films that fall under the category of what can be called 'national cinema', as films that reflect the culture of a specific national group. Post-colonial African cinema has been described by David Murphy and Patrick Williams as an example of national cinema as it addresses questions of national and cultural identity and contributes towards a revision of national history through the recording of colonial atrocities and the recollection and restoration of collective memories.[36]

---

35 Ibid., 10–24.
36 David Murphy and Patrick Williams, *Postcolonial African Cinema* (Manchester: Manchester UP, 2007), 63.

The deconstruction of existing conventions through form rather than through content is an approach that is, while being more marginal, particularly well suited to give expression to traumatic experiences since it reflects the disrupted state of the trauma-impaired memory. I will therefore discuss two examples in greater detail: the French Post-War theatrical productions that have been labelled by Martin Esslin as 'Theatre of the Absurd' and 'Butoh' a modern Japanese dance form that emerged as a response to the bombing of Hiroshima and Nagasaki.

According to Esslin, the 'Theatre of the Absurd' emerged after World War II as an 'unmediated response of independent authors to a disintegrating world that had lost its unifying principle'.[37] For Esslin, the development of this kind of theatre was informed by an intention to express the experience of trauma.[38] The sudden out-of-context occurrence of the trauma memory, the illogical and out-of-character behaviour of the traumatised person, the repetitive and cyclical nature of trauma re-enactments and the general unrelatedness between the individual, his or her actions and the social environment, contain elements of absurdity that are mirrored and expressed by the 'Theatre of the Absurd'. Poetic imagery is used rather than intellectual concepts and the impression of absurdity is created in a variety of ways. This includes action that is unmotivated and nonsensical, a structure that is circular or contains repetitive and circular elements, the use of disjointed clues that don't fit into a meaningful pattern, the lack of any generally accepted value system and the disintegration and devaluation of language.[39]See Figure 10.1 overleaf for a visual example.

As a format that developed in Japan in response to the experience of collective trauma caused by the bombing of Hiroshima and Nagasaki, Butoh is a contemporary dance form that is inspired by German Expressionist theatre. According to Paula Marie Orlando it is also rooted in Japanese cultural history and incorporates elements of Shintoism, Zen Buddhism and images of Japanese cultural life. Deconstructing the conventions of Japanese traditional dance as well as classical Western ballet and in this way rejecting the imperialist concepts by which both were informed, Butoh explores the dark, primordial and subconscious part of the national psyche, giving it the ability to express an 'awakening to mortality and human suffering'.[40] According to Orlando, Butoh is based on a trust on the body's own visceral impulses and allows movements

37 Martin Esslin, *The Theatre of the Absurd* (London: Penguin Books, 1961), 411, 419.

38 Ibid., 414.

39 Ibid., 402, 406, 412, 413, 415.

40 Paula Marie Orlando, 'Cutting the Surface of the Water: Butoh as Traumatic Awakening,' *Social Semiotics* 11.3 (2001), 309.

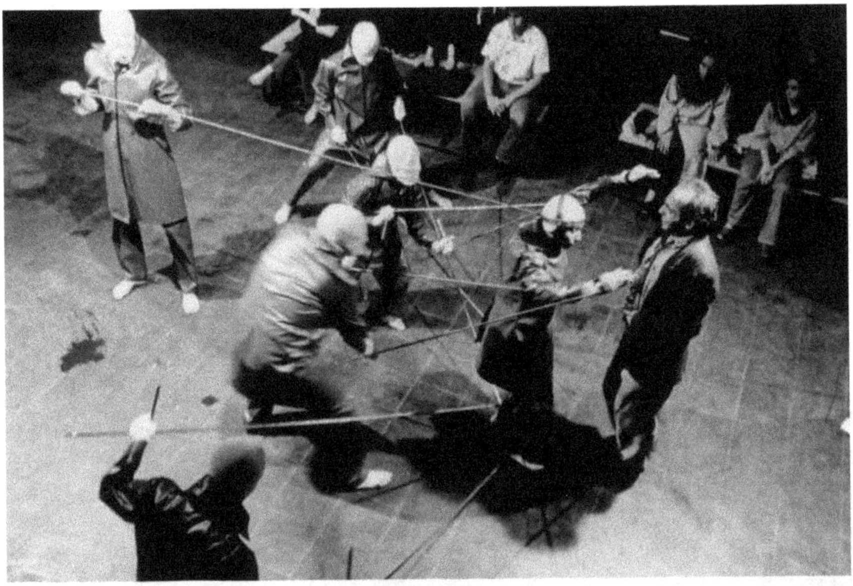

FIGURE 10.1 *Rhinoceros*, by Eugene Ionesco performed by Naqshineh Theatre
COPYRIGHT: IN PUBLIC DOMAIN.

to emerge that reflect the displaced and traumatized self. Orlando sees the Butoh dancer as a metaphor for the survivor. The dancer appears disturbingly vulnerable and without identity. The body is covered in white body paint, the head is either shaved or topped with a wig, movements are minute and slow, gestures are spasmodic, the face is contorted while the sets are starkly illuminated and minimalist. According to Orlando, Butoh reflects, in contrast to classical ballet, a downwards movement, representing 'the fall' and thereby creating a 'body metaphor' for trauma.[41] The deconstruction of established structures is balanced through Butoh's connection to ancient cultural traditions and the return to primordial forms of gesture and movement reintegrates the identity of the traumatised self. Butoh can therefore be experienced as authentic as well as therapeutic. According to Don McLeod, it is due to Butoh's creatively liberating effect that its principles are used in theatre as well as in dance and movement-based therapy internationally today.[42] See Figure 10.2 above for a visual example.

41 Ibid., 317.

42 David McLeod, 'History of Butoh,' (2002), viewed 18 August 2009, http://www.zenbutoh.com/history.htm.

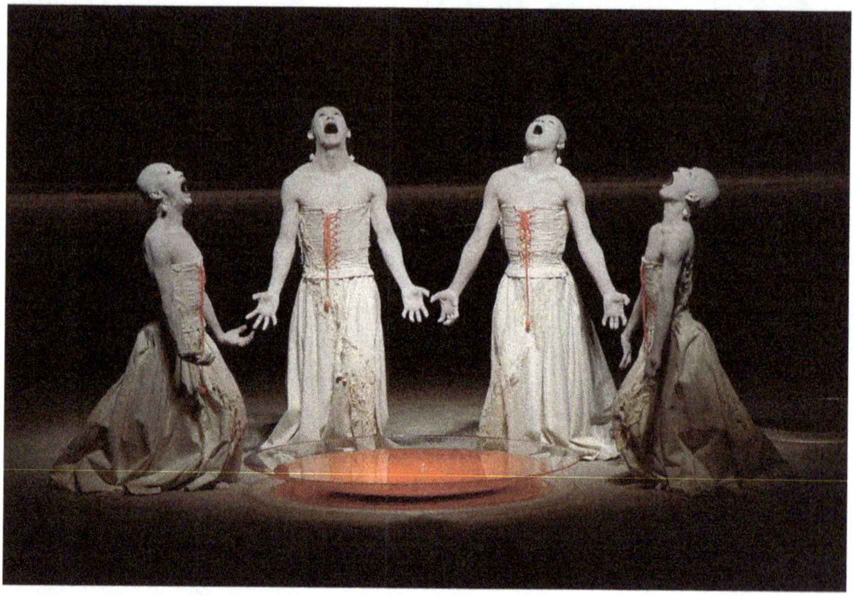

FIGURE 10.2 *Sankai Juku: "HIBIKI – Resonance from Far Away"*
© AKIRA OGATA. CO-PRODUCED BY THEATRE DE LA VILLE, PARIS, FRANCE/ HANCHER AUDITORIUM UNIVERSITY OF IOWA, USA/BIWAKO HALL CENTER FOR THE PERFORMING ARTS SHIGA JAPAN/SANKAI JUKU. WORLD PREMIERED AT THEATRE DE LA VILLE, PARIS IN 1998.

Cultural productions that use a format that deconstructs existing conventional structures like Butoh or what has been labelled by Esslin as the 'theatre of the absurd', can be experienced as challenging and demanding by their audiences and are therefore less widely received than conventional narrative formats. However, it is the active audience engagement that is demanded by those productions that makes the mental and emotional reprocessing that is needed in this context more effective. Rather than being drawn into a conventional narrative structure with its predetermined emotional cues, the audience is confronted with a picture of disintegration, and asked to make 'an active effort towards integration'.[43]

8 A History of Lost Connection

An understanding of trauma as a rupture to our sense of connectivity, be it on the individual, micro- or macro-social level, shows the need for a process that

43 Esslin, *Theatre of the Absurd*, 412–413.

restores the lost sense of connection especially since this rupture can perpetuate itself by furthering conflict and violence.

While each experience of rupture needs to be addressed, it is of vital importance to highlight that we live in a society that is based on a perspective in which a sense of interrelatedness has been lost, which creates a climate that facilitates violence and ongoing traumatisation. This lost sense of connection can be traced through European history to a quotation by Aristotle that shows a perception of humanity as split into two unequal groups, those that are born to rule and those that are born to subjection:

> From this it follows that even warfare is by nature a form of acquisition – for the art of hunting is part of it – which is applied against wild animals and against those men who are not prepared to be ruled, even though they are born to subjection, in so far as this war is just by nature.[44]

The loss of connection is here a fear-based perspective that sees inequality as a given, natural state, thereby legitimising violence. According to Benjamin Isaac, it was this perspective that facilitated the concept of Imperialism that was subsequently adapted and applied by the Romans.[45] Due to the extensive and continuous influence of Graeco-Roman culture, it was this view that fostered hierarchical social stratification, colonialism as well as the relentless struggle for supremacy in Europe.

Julia Smith describes how the Roman Imperial culture continued to affect the European population even after its demise in 500 AD. Having developed from Roman imperial provinces into independent separate kingdoms the civilisation of medieval Europe combined, according to Smith, regional diversity and localism with the many aspects of the cultural, religious and political inheritance of the old empire.[46] Smith describes how a male-centred hierarchical structure was promoted through the implementation of Roman law that legally favoured adult men over minors and women:[47]

> As kings, magnates and bishops it was men who legislated, revised social norms, passed sentence. It was mostly they, or their subordinates, who copied charters, wrote histories and chronicles, composed moral

---

44 Aristotle in Benjamin H. Isaac, 'Proto-Racism in Graeco-Roman Antiquity,' *World Archaeology* 38.1 (2006), 40.

45 Isaac, 'Proto-Racism in Graeco-Roman Antiquity,' 40.

46 Julia M. H. Smith, *Europe after Rome* (Oxford: Oxford UP, 2005), 254, 296, 297.

47 Ibid., 121.

> treatises, delineated ideal social relationships. Legal, intellectual, and religious tradition inherited from the Roman world provided powerful justification for a world tilted in their favour.[48]

A reference to an imagined and mythical past further legitimised privileged local, political and economic positions and restrictions of authority and ensured the continuous transmission of power among the male ruling elite.[49] Smith refers to the instrumental role of Christianity that, once institutionalised and established as state religion, transmitted and preserved Roman culture. The Latin bible contributed in the process by enforcing the concept of imperialism through its references to many ancient empires of which Rome was portrayed as the most recent. As a consequence the term 'empire' was widely employed to describe forms of cultural, political and military domination, and imperial practices were used to display power and enhance legitimacy.[50] The power and influence of both Rome and the church increased further with the installation of a papal monarchy in Rome, which started in the 11th and continued into the 13th century. Smith describes how the papal monarchy eradicated all still persisting forms of local diversities by subjecting the European population to its centralised judicial and administrative authority.[51] The church maintained, according to Smith, its dominant position in early medieval society through the acquisition of land, capital and treasures as well as by securing ideological support. It was therefore in a position to influence and affect social structures and to further social, political, economic as well as gender related stratification.

> It (the church) called for a reordering of daily life, sexual relationships, and family bonds. Its language, technologies of power, cosmology, and far-flung web of contacts together sharpened distinctions of status and gender to foster new, steeply graduated hierarchies of power, at whose apex were rulers whose wealth, power, and prestige lacked precedent in those localities. It promoted the emergence of new imperial polities.[52]

That the oppressive and hierarchical social structures persisted is apparent in Brendan Simms' observations of 'socio-legal inequality' among the European

---

48 Ibid., 147.

49 Ibid., 261, 262.

50 Ibid., 262, 263, 273, 276.

51 Ibid., 293, 294.

52 Ibid., 295.

population in the 18th century. Simms describes a social structure that was based on domination and obligation within the German principalities, where both rural and urban communities were highly stratified and polarized.[53]

It becomes hereby clear how the lost sense of connection that had informed Aristotle's statement and enabled the concept of Imperialism led, through the incorporation of the Graeco-Roman culture into the institutionalised Christian faith, to the establishment of oppressive hierarchical societies in Europe. The fact that these hierarchical societies were based on humiliation and servitude shows that experiences of lost connection can perpetuate themselves indefinitely if they are not addressed in such a way that a reconnection is facilitated.

The concept of imperialism also furthered a continuous struggle for hegemony in Europe. This struggle was particularly intense between France and the German speaking principalities and informed the Thirty Years War, The Napoleonic Invasion and the Prussian War of Liberation, The Franco-Prussian War as well as World War I and World War II.[54] A pattern of humiliation and counter-humiliation as described by Lindner is apparent in this context and particularly obvious in the crowning of the German Kaiser at the Palais de Versailles in 1871 after the German victory over France, meant to spite the French foe. This humiliation was countered by the French in the harsh conditions of the Treaty of Versailles at the end of World War I. Lindner states that the conditions of the treaty were experienced as degrading and humiliating by the defeated German population, which thereby became susceptible to warmongering propaganda. She compares the much more recent genocidal killings that were instigated by Hutu leaders that stirred up fears in their followers about acts of humiliation supposedly planned by their Tutsi neighbours and National Socialist propaganda that portrayed Jews as wanting to enslave all gentiles. In both cases it was the fear of humiliation by those that had previously been humiliated that lead to violent conflict.[55] Lindner's research shows that leaders who appropriate feelings of humiliation are often former victims of humiliation themselves, who driven by their own obsessive urges for retaliation force a population into dichotomies of 'either friend or enemy'. She explains how this process of polarisation fosters a social climate of extremism and prevents criticism, as critics are accused of siding with the 'enemy'. The violation of moral codes therefore goes unpunished, leading to an increase in impunity

---

53 Brendan Simms, *The Struggle for Mastery in Germany 1779–1850* (London: Macmillan Press Ltd, 1998), 19, 20.

54 Kurt F. Reinhardt, *Germany: 2000 Years* (California: The Bruce Publishing Company, 1950), 290, 323.

55 Lindner, 'Healing the Cycles of Humiliation,' 128, 129.

that promotes and facilitates atrocities.[56] The link between a loss of connection, which is here the experience of humiliation and violence that can occur on an individual as well as a societal level simultaneously, is particularly clear in this context.

9 The Need for a Revised Perspective

The urgent need for a revision of the fear-based perspective that legitimises violence becomes apparent, having traced the loss of a sense of connection and its destructive consequences within European history. Since this fear-based perception is at the base of our Western society and informs our thinking on many levels, it is a fundamental rethinking that is called for. Language as an expression of our way of thinking can be instrumental in this process and a revision of its use can become a vehicle for change. Marshall B. Rosenberg developed an alternative model of communication in relation to both speaking and listening that can facilitate such a change. Rosenberg identifies disconnection in the context of communication when speakers trigger feelings like fear, guilt and shame in their listeners through moralistic judgements and static generalisation. He calls this mode of communication 'life-alienating' and proposes a model that fosters reconnection to the self and others as both a remedy and an alternative. He calls this model 'Nonviolent Communication' or NVC.[57] Rosenberg believes that it is an essential part of human nature to give and receive compassionately and that a sense of disconnection from ourselves and others has been caused by what he calls 'destructive cultural learning'.[58] NVC undoes this destructive learning by teaching observation without judgement or evaluation and an ability to apply this form of observation to the action of others, to one's own personal feelings, and to the needs that inform those feelings.[59] Fostering both awareness as well as empathy NVC enables participants to make clear and concrete requests that reflect their own feelings and needs while listening empathetically to the needs of others, thereby facilitating a successful negotiation:

> NVC guides us in reframing how we express ourselves and hear others. Instead of habitual, automatic reactions, our words become conscious

56 Ibid., 134.

57 Marshall B. Rosenberg, *Nonviolent Communication: a Language of Life* (Encinitas, Ca: PuddleDancer Press, 2003), 17, 20.

58 Ibid., 171.

59 Ibid., 6, 7.

> responses based firmly on awareness of what we are perceiving, feeling and wanting. We are led to express ourselves with honesty and clarity, while simultaneously paying others a respectful and empathetic attention.[60]

Rosenberg holds that life-alienating communication reflects and re-enforces hierarchical social structures and that a communication that encourages a re-connection between the self and the other can also contribute towards social change:

> Life-alienating communication both stems from and supports hierarchical and domination societies, where large populations are controlled by small numbers of individuals to those individuals own benefit … the language of wrongness, should and have to, is perfectly suited to this purpose: the more people are trained to think in terms of moralistic judgements that imply wrongness and badness, the more they are trained to look outside themselves – to outside authorities – for the definition of what constitutes right, wrong, good and bad. When we are in contact with our feelings and needs, we humans no longer make good slaves and underlings.[61]

10 Conclusion

In the preceding pages I have argued that trauma causes a sense of disruption to our predisposition towards interconnectivity and that this loss of connection can perpetuate itself by causing violence which causes further trauma and disconnection. This pattern that can also be observed in the social context, can be traced through history to a perspective that sees inequality as natural and violence as legitimate. Being at the base of our Western society, it is this world-view that has enabled hierarchical and dominant social structures to become established, thereby perpetuating the traumatic effect of lost interconnectedness in the macro-social context. To restore our lost sense of connection to ourselves as well as to others this perspective needs to be called into question. The revised perspective has to be based on a raised awareness that supports what Rosi Braidotti calls an ethics of 'sustainable affirmative relations'[62] which

60 Ibid., 3.

61 Ibid., 23.

62 Rosi Braidotti, *Transpositions: On Nomadic Ethics* (Cambridge: Polity Press, 2006), 209.

facilitates the recognition and renegotiation of our being 'in this together',[63] leading towards 'the construction of communities where the notion of transience, of passing is acknowledged in a sober secular manner that binds us to the multiple 'others' in a vital web of interrelations'.[64]

While providing a simple and practical method that can help to establish such a perspective, Rosenberg also acknowledged how challenging and difficult this process is, since it comprises a fundamental revision of all that we have learnt so far:

> [D]estructive cultural learning ... is so ingrained in our lives that we are no longer conscious of it. In the same way, pain engendered by damaging cultural conditioning is such an integral part of our lives that we can no longer distinguish its presence. It takes tremendous energy and awareness to recognize this destructive learning and to transform it into thoughts and behaviors that are of value and of service to life.[65]

Confronting trauma and its effects in such a way that acknowledges the loss of connection and promotes increased awareness can be an important step in this direction leading us 'home' towards a restoration of our initial ability for compassionate interaction. Trauma and trauma-like experiences can in this way become valuable opportunities for growth and learning.

> We need future-oriented perspectives, which do not deny the traumas of the past but transform them into possibilities for the present.[66]

Bibliography

Alexander, Jeffrey C. 'Towards a Theory of Cultural Trauma.' *Cultural Trauma and Collective Identity*, Jeffrey C. Alexander, Ron Eyerman, Bernhard Giesen, Neil J. Smelser, Piotr Sztompka, 1–30. California: UP Berkeley, 2004.

Bergmann, Uri. 2008 'Further thoughts on the Neurobiology of EMDR: The Role of the Cerebellum in Accelerated Information Processing.' *Traumatology* 6 (2000), 175–200.

Braidotti, Rosi. *Transpositions: On Nomadic Ethics*. Cambridge: Polity Press, 2006.

63 Ibid., 228.
64 Ibid., 271.
65 Rosenberg, *Nonviolent Communication*, 171.
66 Braidotti, Transpositions, 268.

Collins, Randall. *Interaction Ritual Chains*. Princeton NJ: Princeton UP, 2004.

Collins, Randall. *Violence*. Princeton NJ: Princeton UP, 2008.

Esslin, Martin. *The Theatre of the Absurd*. London: Penguin Books, 1961.

Giddens, Anthony. *Social Theory and Modern Sociology*. Stanford: Stanford UP, 1987.

Isaac, Benjamin H. 'Proto-Racism in Graeco-Roman Antiquity.' *World Archaeology* 38.1 (2006): 32–47.

Kandel, Eric. *In Search of Memory*. New York: Norton & Company Inc, 2006.

LeDoux, Joseph. *The Synaptic Self*. New York: Penguin Books Ltd, 2002.

LeDoux, Joseph. *The Emotional Brain*. New York: Simon and Schuster Paperbacks, 1996.

Levine, Peter. *Healing Trauma*. Boulder Co: Sounds True Inc, 2005.

Levine, Peter. 'Nature's Lesson in Healing Trauma' (1997). Viewed 26 January 2013. http://traumahealing.com/somatic-experiencing/reference-healing-trauma-lessons-from-nature.pdf.

Lewis, Helen. *Shame and Guilt in Neurosis*. New York: IUP, 1971.

Lindner, Evelin Gerda. 'Healing the Cycles of Humiliation: How to Attend to Emotional Aspects of "Unsolvable Conflicts" and the Use of "Humiliation Entrepreneurship," ' *Peace and Conflict*, Journal of Peace Psychology, 8.2 (2002), 125–138.

Lisak, David. 'The Neurobiology of Trauma' (unpublished article 2002). Viewed 29 August 2009. http://www.nowldef.org/html/njep/dvd/pdf/neurobiology.pdf.

McLeod, David. 'History of Butoh,' (2002). Viewed 18 August 2009. http://www.zenbutoh.com/history.htm.

Moore, Robert H. 'Background and theory of Traumatic Incident Reduction.' *Traumatic Incident Reduction: Research and results* edited by Volkmann V. R., 15–17. Michigan: Loving Healing Press, 2005.

Mosse, George. *The Crisis of German Ideology*. New York: Schoken Books, 1964.

Murphy, David and Patrick Williams. *Postcolonial African Cinema.* Manchester: Manchester UP, 2007.

Nairn, Thomas. *The Break-up of Britain*. London: New Left Books, 1977.

Orlando, Paula Marie. 'Cutting the Surface of the Water: Butoh as Traumatic Awakening.' *Social Semiotics* 11.3 (2001): 307–324.

Pulzer, Peter. *Germany 1870–1945*. Oxford: Oxford UP 1997.

Reinhardt, Kurt F. *Germany: 2000 Years.* California: The Bruce Publishing Company, 1950.

Rosenberg, Marshall B. *Nonviolent Communication: a Language of Life*. Encinitas, Ca: PuddleDancer Press, 2003.

Scaer, Robert. 'The Neurobiology of Dissociation and Chronic Disease' *Applied Psychophysiology and Biofeedback* 26.1 (2009): 73–91.

Scheff, Thomas. 'Theory of Runaway Nationalism: Love of Country/Hatred of Others' (FPR-UCLA Interdisciplinary conference: *The Seven Dimensions of Emotions,* University of California Los Angeles, 30th March – 1st April 2007, unpublished manuscript). Viewed 8 March 2009. http://www.soc.ucsb.edu/faculty/scheff.

Simms, Brendan. *The struggle for Mastery in Germany 1779–1850*. London: Macmillan Press Ltd, 1998.

Smith, Julia M. H. *Europe after Rome*. Oxford: Oxford UP, 2005.

van der Kolk, Bessel A. 'Developmental Trauma Disorder,' *Psychiatric Annals*, 35.5 (2005), 2.

Index of Subjects

Index of Modern Authors

www.ingramcontent.com/pod-product-compliance
Lightning Source LLC
Chambersburg PA
CBHW071441230926
51846CB00001B/307
9789004350809